# Recommendations

"*Pure pleasure...*

"This book, that is precisely appropriate for the times we live in, is an important and educational journey towards greater self-awareness, health, the formation of clarity and independence and opening up to new horizons.

"This book provides a light, funny and interesting breakdown of the psychological complexes in our life in an unusual way which interweaves rich imagery, analogies and fundamental insights. It provides mechanisms of action which enable every individual to make significant changes in his life, to be his own psychologist, to grow up and develop into a modality of existence which is fundamentally different."

-- **Sharon Gal,** a holistic psychotherapist, a companion in processes of development and acceleration in accordance with New Age values.

"In this book, the author offers paths of deep, honest and accessible self-reflection. As a psychotherapist, I found considerable interest in this book since people who undergo psychological therapy require intense and laborious internal work and inner reflections without which the work of the most skilled therapist will be for naught. In other words, work on a deep and significant commitment requires internal reflection and assuming complex personal responsibility -- even if you have a therapist to guide you through the process. In her clear and fluent writing, Meirav offers "milestones" that expand the scope and the toolbox of the therapy. Even experienced therapists will benefit from this book, gaining a better understanding of the depths of their patient's souls and a broader and more creative perspective."

-- **Sigal Tzach**, Psychotherapist MSW, dynamic therapy of adults.

"The book is interesting, fascinating and written in easily understood language. It comes in the midst of a period in which interest is increasing, both among the general public and in the medical world, regarding the complex and incompletely understood relationship between body and soul, its impact and implications on our physical and mental health. This book adds to this mixture an additional layer which offers an entirely different perspective.

"This book will speak to and contribute both to people who are aware of the body-soul-spirit trilogy and to those people who have yet to be exposed to the metaphysical layer of life. The book can enrich the average person by increasing his understanding of his emotional-psychological processes and by initiating processes of change. For those who are already undergoing various therapeutic processes, this book has the potential of better clarifying and improving the therapist mediated process."

-- **Dr. Aaron Alexandrovitz**, an internal medicine specialist, a psychotherapist and a lecturer at Tel Aviv University Medical School

How to Be Our Own Psychologists?
Meirav Harel



Translation from the Hebrew: Jonathan Boxman
Contact: meirav.harel1@gmail.com

ISBN 9781984974099

# How to Be Our Own
# PSYCHOLOGISTS?

## MEIRAV HAREL

# Contents

# Acknowledgements

I wish to thank all of the spiritual teachers who accompanied me on the personal level and who taught, reminded, emphasized, guided, transformed, cleaned, empowered and supported me throughout my personal journey of development which eventually also led me to write this book: Daphna Rosenshtok, Dr. Shoshana Zimmerman, Dr. Yael Yisraelov, Ronit Shefi Wolfin and beloved Lou harya, who is a living pillar of fire to all of us. Thanks as well to the male of the pack, Michael Assedo. In addition to the mentors I personally met, my deep and abiding thanks to the many thousands of wise masters who have walked beneath this sun from ancient days to modern times and who have transmitted some small part of their wisdom, spiritual perspective and courage to me, be it through ancient scriptures or YouTube lectures.

I also want to thank Dr. Shaul Tal, Chairman of the Focus Publishing Company, for his boundless generosity and providing me with a professional and high quality home for my books as well as for the rest of the Focus Team for their open hearts, attentiveness, kindness and professionalism.

# Preface

By Dr. **Tomer Sivron**

Meirav Harel's book, "How to Be Our Own Psychologists?" is an important and excellent book which will help anyone who reads it to live a more liberated and love- and life-filled life. In the book, Meirav sketches a map of life and our existence in this world. The reader is presented with a multi-dimensional map which can help him both understand his place in the world and in life and aid him to navigate his way to wherever he wishes to reach.

Meirav has developed an ordered system which she calls "the trilogy method." She presents it to the reader in clear and flowing language, scattering a great deal of humor into the instruction which makes the reading experience easier and lighter. The book also contains a great deal of information that expands and enriches the consciousness and awareness of the reader.

Suffering is an inseparable part of life, but pain is also a guide that can be used to release ourselves from burdensome beliefs and internal bonds so that we can live a life with reduced suffering. Meirav shows us, in this magnificent book, step-by-step, how to release ourselves from suffering and use it to develop to higher and better places.

Meirav assists the reader in developing an attitude of

acceptance and compassion towards oneself and an understanding that we are doing the best that we can at any given moment – "That is the best I can do as of this time point. Perhaps tomorrow I will be able to do more or the day after or next week and perhaps only in a year. Right now, this is my best" – is one of the milestones which Meirav presents to the reader. There are many more of them.

Meirav shares her personal story with the reader detailing how she freed herself from addictions and other harmful and destructive patterns. By doing so she shows that it is indeed possible to change aspects of one's life and that every situation is an opportunity for growth and empowerment. Her exciting personal story, as well as many other examples interwoven in the book, grant the reader the feeling of authenticity and reliability. It is real and it works.

Meirav's book comes precisely at a time when our world is crying out for change and people are seeking alternative ways to cure their bodies and themselves. Many are undergoing a process of awakening and understanding that body and matter are only one pillar of who and what we are and that we are, in fact, much more than that. The understanding that the "external is a reflection of the internal" is critical to assuming responsibility for our lives and to the understanding that we are the only ones who can change our life and ourselves. Others can help, support, direct – but we are the ones who need to make the change and do the work. Meirav's book does exactly that.

To summarize, I warmly recommend Meirav's book. It will contribute to anyone who reads it, whatever his worldview might be. I would also like to thank Meirav for her contribution through her writing.

With love,

**Tomer Sivron**

Clinical-spiritual therapist with a Ph. D. in neurobiology, lecturer and writer. Author of *Turning the Wheel* -- A Journey from Injury to Growth, *Wake Up! A Practical-Spiritual Guide* and *Meeting God at the Stoplight.*

# Introduction

We all face challenges in our life. We all get slapped down by life. We all get stuck at some point or another in our lives. We get stuck in places that are not necessarily good for us. We get stuck with people that don't necessarily desire or promote our well-being (be they bosses, friends or acquaintances) or else we get stuck in situations which we don't know how to get out of and which we are, perhaps, even afraid to deal with. This is part of life and it happens to the best of us.

One of the reasons it might be difficult for us to pull free of where we are stuck is that too many emotions (both open and hidden) are involved. This emotional mix makes it difficult for us to consider matters clearly or rationally and sometimes even deliberately blinds us. If we go to a psychologist or a therapist, it is likely that he can provide us with the perspective which emotional detachment enables. Later on, depending on our level of exposure, maturity and preparedness, light may even be shed on several optional mechanisms of dealing with the situation, both on the emotional-psychological level and the mental-consciousness level, in order to help us extract ourselves from the obstruction where we are stuck and even leverage it for personal development.

What happens when we cannot afford professional therapy, whether due to either economic reasons (I can't afford it), unavailability (I don't have time for this), shame (there is no way that I am sharing personal information with a stranger), despair (none of this will help me / there is no way to change the situation), various other fears (there are so many charlatans in the field of therapy / I don't feel like opening up a Pandora's box) or reasons of non-awareness (this is just a waste of money / why even bother poking around in the past? What is done is done and over with).

The trilogy method for analyzing and extracting ourselves from these obstructions is a diagnostic tool I developed during my work in a clinic with people who desired to make a change in their lives or else cure themselves of diseases or chronic pains. It does not presume to be a substitute for professional treatment. However, if we cannot, at a given point in our lives, get the support of professional help, this system can certainly help us help ourselves -- even if only on the level of urgent "first aid" -- by providing us with a highly intellectual perspective that will enable us to examine the situation and interpret it from a slightly different perspective than we are familiar with. This perspective will enable us to make a change. It might even reverse how we think and feel about this situation. This change certainly has the power to initiate movement towards moving past the obstruction where we are stuck.

The trilogy method helps enable diagnosing and leaving these obstructions behind. It can be treated as reading glasses – glasses that we put on only when we want to read and remove once we are done. We do not keep these reading glasses on all day long because we see well enough without them. But, when we want to read something and we can't see what is written because the letters are blurred or out of focus, then we need to put the reading glasses on and, in a single magical second, they help us see and understand what is written.

This is what the trilogy method is. It provides us with the clarifying focus that can enable us to recognize and move past where we are stuck relatively quickly and even experience liberation and / or relief -- if, of course, we choose to implement in practice the insights that we receive and act in accordance to them.

The trilogy method provides us with a significant shortcut and spares us a great deal of headaches, confusion, anger and other such delights -- if we are prepared and capable of honestly answering the three questions that the method asks and courageously meet the changes required by these answers. As is well-known (or perhaps it is not so well-known), there really aren't any shortcuts in life. Each and every one of us has to face the quota of challenges and obstacles life has placed, places and will continue to place in the way. (That is just the way life here on earth is. Hardship and challenges are what makes you learn, internalize and grow the most. For the most part, you only understand this in retrospect -- when they actually occur they are experienced as a depressing difficulty.) However, there are certainly occasional specific situations that require immediate solutions. The trilogy method answers these needs as well. This method can be used in precise-tactical diagnosis to focus and improve the precision of a deeper process or to raise issues whose time has come to be recognized and addressed. This depends, of course, on the specific circumstances, on our openness, on our honesty, on our preparedness and on our readiness to come to terms with the deeper layers of our soul.

This system is based on both known and accepted earthly principles and metaphysical principles which are not quite as known or accepted. Accordingly, for those of us who detest whatever is not perceived by the five senses and / or scientifically proven (proven as of this moment because everything changes all the time), my recommendation is that we resolve to give this system a chance to work for us -- even if we do not agree with all of its premises if only because it is capable of helping us and providing us with a relatively rapid solution to the situation which we are dealing with. Once we achieve that resolution, we can tell all of the voices in our head screaming, "Bullshit /nonsense / unproven / what are you talking about? / Come on," "Ladies and gentlemen, kindly remain seated, take a breather, drink a glass of water and calm down. We are only taking a second to check out what is being offered here and we will be right back. We promise" or "We are only putting on our glasses for a second, taking a look and taking them right back off -- all right?"

Let the results speak for themselves -- have we or have we not, been helped? Have we received a new perspective on the situation? Have we received new insights that have opened up our mind? Have we successfully changed what we think and / or feel about the obstruction we are experiencing and are stuck in? Have we, thanks to our change in thought and emotion, succeeded in changing our actions or behavior in practice? Do we now know how to break free of the obstruction or don't we? Do we know which path leads us forward to the exit?

Instead of mincing further words, have a look at the preliminary presentation of the three parts of the trilogy below. The simplicity of the three questions in the third part may be deceptive. Although you might view them as simple, answering them requires a great deal of courage and precision. Still, if you dare use them, you will certainly receive precise direction regarding the path to follow. This guidance will be synchronized with all of the parts of which you are made, both hidden and apparent. That is just how we are, simple and complex at the same time….

That said, here is the essence of the trilogy method:

1. **The three parts of man**

    I.   The temporal body
    II.  The temporal soul
    III. The eternal spirit

2. **The three premises**

    I.   Opportunities arrive in disguise
    II.  Self-compassion instead of berating ourselves.
    III. Every setback is an opportunity for growth

3. **The three questions**

    I.   Where is the silver lining in the cloud?
    II.  Why did we create the situation?
    III. What can we do to change the situation in thought, emotion and action?

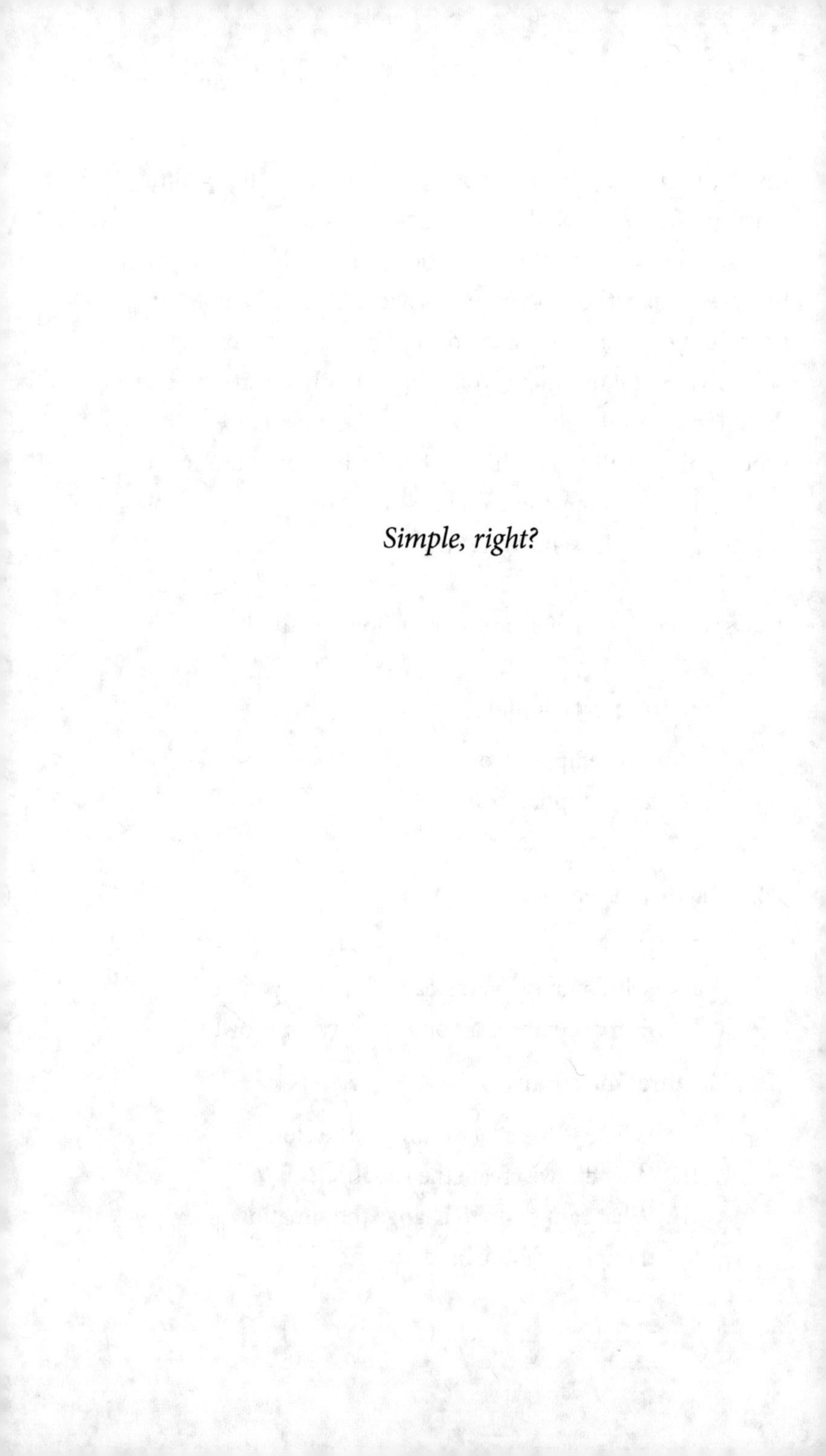

*Simple, right?*

# The Three Parts of Man

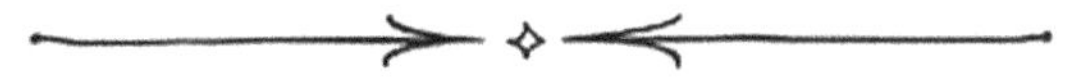

*The temporal body*

*The temporal soul*

*The eternal spirit*

For those for whom this information is new, it is best, at this stage, to simply accept the tripartite nature of man as axiomatic and deal with its ramifications later, in the questions section. There is no need to let what you don't even know get in the way of getting the help you want to get, right? During antiquity, the belief that man was not merely his body nor even his body and soul, but a trilogy of body, soul and the spirit was predominant. Just like a trilogy in the arts where each artistic creation is both an independent creation in its own right and interlinked with the others, so do each of these three components of the human artistic trilogy exist both independently and symbiotically with each other. It is within this trilogy that the parts communicate, both openly and clandestinely, consciously and subconsciously. Indeed, they constantly exchange data on many levels (physical-biological and biochemical, psychological-emotional, mental-consciousness and metaphysical (everything not picked up by the five known senses) as well as energetic.

## A trilogy of the body, the soul and the spirit

**The body** -- The well-known physical body, the "celebrity" of the trilogy, a super-complex machine in which trillions of cells and an inconceivable number of biochemical activities take place at any given moment in order to ensure the ongoing existence of the human body, without our knowledge aid. It is very good that this is so. Why? Because for the most part, where we are consciously involved (diet and nutrition, lifestyle...), we do a very good job at screwing up and sabotaging ourselves -- even if that is not our desire or intent.

**The soul** -- This is the array of thoughts, perceptions and emotions that define who we are in this existence, who we perceive ourselves to be in this life, both in our consciousness and in our emotional array. The soul is also a celebrity, though a rather "recent" one. It debuted "only" a century or so ago, in the late 19th century, thanks to the groundbreaking work of the Viennese Jew Zigmund-Shlomo, better known to the world as Freud, the founder of modern psychology (Psychology = the study of the psyche = soul.) This soul shares an expiration date with our body-- when one ceases to exist, so does the other. Both are temporal. Both share the same "terminal illness" all humans suffer -- from the moment we are born, the countdown to death begins and there are no exceptions.

**The spirit** -- This is the new kid on the block, the child of the New Age, at least insofar as the supposedly enlightened and technologically advanced Western Society is concerned. In contrast, the spirit has starred in many ancient civilizations all over the world and was the subject of much admiration and respect. Since the dawn of humanity, many have tried to define this eternal, divine part present in each human being. It was defined by many names -- essence, the divine spark, the higher self and so on. In this book we will refer to it simply as the spirit. This is, without a doubt, the part hardest to explain or even acknowledge since those lucky enough to actually experience it and receive proof that something is left of us after we breathe our last breath, are those who died clinical deaths. In other words, died ["and the dust returns to the earth as it was and the spirit returns to God who gave it." (**Ecclesiastes: 12: 7**)] and then returned to tell the tale.

There are tens of thousands of recorded incidents of clinical death from all over the world. These incidents include individuals of all ages, genders, religions and cultures. Indeed, a poll held in 1992 by Gallup indicated that the number of people in the United States alone who experienced clinical death and survived was 13 million out of a population of 260 million -- 5% of the population. Just imagine how many people worldwide must have experienced the phenomenon!

What all of the recorded experiences have in common is the description by the individuals (including little children), of their consciousness leaving their cramped body and expanding into an existence that is independent of time, space or the physical laws known to this world. We will not go into questions such as: "What are the worlds they visited? What and who did they see there? What did they feel? What did they learn there about themselves or the world? Why did they have this experience to begin with?" Know, however, that these stories are fascinating and exciting. I recommended you sample them; they will touch your soul.[1]

Fine. So, 5% of us received direct proof and know for sure that there is some sort of consciousness that continues to exist even after the death of the physical body. Good for them. No, really. Congratulations and best of wishes, but what about the rest of us? All the other 95%? All the regular Joes who never died and then came back to tell the tale? All those who are still "scared to death" of the inconceivable and seemingly unfair non-existence that awaits them -- even if they carefully suppress this fear in their everyday life?

We can get a small sample of what it means to exist "independently of time or space" every night, when we dream.

---

1        Recommended literature on the topic of clinical death as written by physicians includes: 'Beyond Death's Door' by Dr. Morris Rollings, "On Death and Dying" by Dr. Elizabeth Kovler-Ross, "Life after Death" by Dr. Raymond Murray, "The Light Beyond" by Dr. Michael Sabom and "Evidence of the Afterlife: The Science of Near-Death Experiences" by Dr. Jeffery Long. All can be purchased through Amazon.

(Who hasn't experienced flying like a bird or swimming like a fish in a dream? Or being several places at the same time? Or skipping between different periods in a single dream?) When we dream, our waking mind is completely shut down and is snoring away peacefully and yet we remain conscious on some level. We are aware of everything that happens to us in the dream, we know who is with us, what we see, what we say and even what we feel but we feel all this when our body and soul are asleep. In other words, **we are not conscious and yet a consciousness still exists**. The consciousness we experience in a dream is a sample, however small, of the sensation we can experience and the closest we can get to the eternal consciousness that lives on after our body and our soul complete their role and return to dust. This is the spirit, the eternal essence within us that is not dependent on time or space.

So what do we have? A single human being made up of three parts living under the same roof, two which are temporal and one which is eternal. It is not at all simple to live this way. There are disagreements, conflicts, claims, demands, goals, needs and desires which are mostly unsynchronized and even contradictory, mostly because the two temporal "celebrities" are almost completely unaware of the existence of the eternal part which is usually hidden.

## Where is the coach really headed?

There is ancient imagery regarding the relationship between the three parts which likens man to a coach in motion. The coach and the horses are the physical body, the coachman is the soul and a hidden passenger deep within the coach is the spirit.[2] The horses and the coach, the physical body, must be cared for with food, water, rest, cleanliness and maintenance so they can ride in the most optimal manner. The coachman, the soul, has both physical needs and thoughts, emotions, desires and needs (conscious and unconscious). It is he who is the driver of the coach and it is he who decides where the destination is. Or at least so he thinks. Why? Because the person actually controlling the destination is the hidden passenger, of whom the coachman is not even aware. That hidden passenger has the ability to implant thoughts in the mind of the coachman and in that way he transmits to him the destinations he himself wishes to reach. However, even when those destinations are transmitted from the hidden passenger to the coachman, and he experiences them as his own thoughts, the hidden passenger will not always have his way. The coachman might deviate from those destinations or not reach them according to the time that the hidden passenger desires. He might suddenly decide to stop for a pint or two at a pub because the road is boring and filled with potholes and the bumpy ride is driving him nuts. Alternatively, perhaps he might run into an interesting group of people who are traveling elsewhere and feel like joining them. Maybe he even runs into a beautiful woman on the way, who happens to be traveling in the opposite direction. You get the analogy right?

---

2       I was introduced to this analogy by my spiritual mentor, Dr. Shoshana Zimmerman.

The point is that there is considerable interaction between many desires, both apparent and hidden, that sometimes work in concert and, at other times, are completely unrelated.

## Opposing perspectives

Another way of looking at this fascinating and complex trilogy that makes up each and every one of us is through the perspective of each of the parts and their different goals. *The perspective of the spirit is above all eternal-immortal* so it simply is not wrapped up, as our conscious and unconscious mind tends to be, with the hourglass of our life trickling away. This means that it is not motivated by pressure. It always was and always will be just like the definition of energy, inexhaustible but capable of transforming. *Its perspective is extremely distant and it looks at life from a bird's-eye viewpoint.* This enables it to see the full picture, including all the data and details that are not apparent at that time point and the adjusted calculation of all of that data. Furthermore, *the perspective of the spirit relates to the lessons we are here to learn* during the sequence of our life's events and what would encourage the best and most powerful growth and development. Therefore, it is generally wiser and more intelligent than the soul which mostly sees only what is right in front of it and only what it faces in its daily life, at a specific time point, simply because it lacks the ability to see further or to include data from the past into the given present.

The perspective of the soul is temporal, perishing and "one-time." It is *mostly focused on survival* (thanks to the millions of lions, tigers and bears that preyed upon prehistoric man) and *ego driven*. The ego originally had a very positive role in safeguarding us from injury and motivating us to accomplishment but it has a tendency to dominate and disrupt our balance (the ego has an ego) which can cloud our perception. Just as importantly, the soul is linked to a physical body that has its own animal needs and desires which sometimes, during a period of extreme scarcity (of food or sex for example), make the man no more than a beast or a bestial man. How can one make reasoned, intelligent decisions from this bestial position? It is impossible or at least very difficult to "function properly" under these conditions.

## The spirit as a navigation app

Another aspect of the perspective of the spirit is that it operates on the foundation of *cosmic, non-linear and interdependent time where everything occurs simultaneously, in parallel, without distinction between past, present and future and without any time-space limitations.* Since we do not really understand what "everything happens simultaneously without any limitations of time or space" means, I will try to provide an analogy that might slightly clarify this challenging idea. In this analogy, we compare the perspective and functions of the spirit to a navigation application such as Waze. We use it when we are on the roads and wish to reach our destination in the fastest and shortest way. The application *knows what our destination is,* including points on the way if we specified such, and it offers us, after it *incorporates additional data in its calculations* such as traffic, accidents on the way or road-work, a number of optimal paths. We pick one and are on our way. The program constantly *tracks* our location and *guides* us every step of the way indicating where we should turn. It *shares* much additional data with us such as where police cars are lying in wait, how long we are expected to be stuck in an annoying traffic jam, our ETA, the speed limit on a given road and even what cafes in the area are recommended or where the nearest pharmacy is. If the program recommends we turn left and for one reason or another we turned right, it immediately "recalculates our course" and shows us how to reach our destination from our current location. We can deviate a dozen times from the course it offers us, for example leave Chicago for New York and end up in L.A. and it will still be there for us, offering us a new alternate and optimal route from LA to New York. It is not angry with us, it does not judge us and it does not berate us or punish us. Instead, it just *continues showing us the optimal way to reach our destination* while incorporating all of the various data in the calculation of the optimal path.

One can further say of the emphatic navigation application and also of the spirit that they fulfill a version of a well-known saying by Rabbi Akiva, a second century Jewish religious scholar: "Everything is foreseen, yet free will is given." *The spirit has all the data regarding all the possible routes and it already knows where each one of them leads.* The routes are like rewinds of movies it has already seen and it therefore knows exactly what is going to happen in each and every one of them. (The spirit fulfilling the "everything is foreseen" part.) And yet, the soul may pick whichever route it wishes, change its mind hundreds of time midway and even select a different destination dozens of time. (The soul fulfilling the second section of the saying "yet free will is given.") The application does not interfere in our choices and only offers us the optimal alternative in regard to our location on any given moment, even if that location seems to be a dead end. It will show us how to get out of that dead end and how to reach our destination.

Unlike the spirit, the soul operates in linear time which has a past, a present and a future. One thing leads to another and causality reigns supreme. What has happened has already happened and what has not happened has yet to happen and no one knows what will happen next. In the present, we try to aim at a desirable reality but no one really knows what will happen in practice as the constantly frustrated sport-gambling junkies will testify when the results of the weekly games fail to match their expectations and guesses for that week. I will note, as an aside, that the soul is not infallible. Like many of us, it tends to be fixated ether on the past -- by enabling what occurred a long time ago to continue to affect our decision-making process in the present or the future -- by allowing our ignorance of "what will be?" (fear of the unknown) to affect our experience of the present. This makes us less self-conscious and less invested in the here and now. In other words, cut off from ourselves and / or our environment, which is why our thoughts, feelings and deeds are not necessarily synchronized with what we are and who we really want to be and be with. It is not for nothing that millennia-old spiritual traditions instruct us to *"live the moment."*

All right, let us return to the main discourse.

To summarize this point, if we can return for a moment to the analogy of the spirit as Waze, the navigation application, *our soul in this analogy is the average driver on the road, who only knows what he can see, perhaps a mile under optimal conditions.* The driver can know what lies beyond his field of view only through the use of the Waze application since he has no way of knowing what is happening ten miles away from him or on the other roads in the country or how long it would take him to travel from one unfamiliar place to another unfamiliar point. Whatever is not perceived through one of his five senses (in the physical space where his body is) remains unknown to him at any given moment and therefore his interpretation of the data and the decisions he makes in regard to the rest of the road is *inadequate* or *lacking in higher knowledge.* Not, of course, because he is stupid but simply because he lacks access to *the spirit's higher knowledge.*

## A negative versus positive perspective

We have reached the final point that refers to the differences in the perspectives of the spirit and the soul. All right kids, guess which of the two is positive in its orientation and which is connected to negative emotions, even though, to its credit, far more than it would like and through no fault of its own? Which of the two is enlightened and which walks in darkness? Which of the two tends to automatically react with compassion and grace and which keeps a gun close to hand (almost purely for self-protection of course) 24/7? Which of the two seeks the good and which one keeps on fleeing from evil? Which of the two looks at the half-full glass and which one bitches and whines, usually, about the glass being half-empty? Which of the two experiences unity and which one experiences separation? Well kids, you no doubt guessed correctly which is which, not because you know the spirit and the soul so well but because we associate ourselves all too well with the challenging one, to put it mildly.

If we return for a moment to that 5% of the population who experienced clinical death and then came back to tell other mortals of what they saw and experienced in the netherworld where they were temporary guests, almost all of them describe same general experience of being *immersed within an entity which was very unfamiliar, even alien, to us human beings but was characterized by extraordinary grace, harmony, compassion, love, calm, peace, acceptance and a high intelligence that enables almost automatic understanding of "why things are as they are."* Is it any wonder that many of them reported that they did not want to return from this place of contentment to a reality where their lives were so different, if not opposite, from what they experienced in the next world?

But what about the other 95%, those who were not graced by this sublime symphony, whose soul and hearts were not touched and changed by it? What about the 95% who are stuck in traffic every day, who swelter in global warming and tremble at global terror? A tiny sample of this sublime entity which exists within each and every one of us (even if we can never put it under a microscope to be tested and measured), can be found in extreme disaster-like situations. We excel in them. *When disasters, accidents, wars, conflagrations and other natural disasters occur, the spirit rises out of the depths and most of us go out of our way and break our patterns. We move to a mode of pure giving of attention, of incredible caring and compassion for the other, of supreme goodness, general harmony and the breakdown of the barriers of religion, race and gender that divide humankind from one another.* As I said, we really stand out in these situations, so much so that a viewer can be moved to tears. Moreover, it does not take colossal mega disasters to see this divine spark within us shine out. You can also see it in tiny disasters such as a man who suddenly collapses in the middle of the street. It is this divine spark that impels us to run and assist this man without thinking twice about it.

However, what happens in our everyday life? What happens in the work-traffic jam-nerves-home-traffic jam-mortgage–nerves-children–joy-nerves routine? *In our everyday life, this magical spark no longer takes center stage.* It returns backstage. The spirit retreats back into our depths but its voice is the *small, silent whisper* in the back of our minds that we rarely notice. It does not shout or use amplification. It whispers and it is hard for us to hear it -- because we live in a *loud and chaotic world* bombarded by thousands of messages at any given moment and because we are exhausted by all of the many disappointments life has so generously endowed us with. We shield ourselves with protective walls and dare anyone to try to breach them. *It is hard to hear the small still voice of the spirit when we are hunkered down behind reinforced and soundproofed walls.*

Moreover, our soul, the seat of all our thoughts and emotions, is permanently immersed in a pool of negativity. That is its point of departure in this story called man. If we map and list all of the thoughts running through our head, we will find that the *absolute majority of our thoughts are negative* (and even optimistic and positive people have m-a-n-y negative thoughts). This is hardly surprising given the fact that our brain is programmed from the dawn of time to achieve one supreme purpose -- survival. Even if for thousands of years we were continuously terrified that we would either be eaten or starve to death, today the danger that the local lion or cannibal will crack our bones as an appetizer is close to zero. The only thing that can "eat us alive" is the mortgage. Most of us either physically overeat and / or gorge ourselves on our negative emotions. And yet, the instinct remains, *the existential survival instinct remains and has merely joined us in our relocation* from the open savannas to the steel and concrete urban jungle where most of us live. This survival instinct of our soul is expressed both in fear of our unknown (I better stay where I am even if I'm up to my armpits in shit -- at least I know this shit and it's warm) and in the general feeling that something terrible is at the door, something evil might happen at any moment. You do not need to be a trauma survivor to constantly fear that a potential predator might come knocking at your door and that your home is built on foundations of sand from which you might be uprooted at any moment. *We are all just walking bags of emotional waste that has accumulated all our lives.* And that waste contains guilt, shame, various fears, anger and rage of various types and a great deal of diverse types of pain. Each one of us may contain his own unique dosage and mix of pain, but we are all driven by the same range of negative emotions and *our thoughts, words and actions are driven by them.* Now go live your life with such a starting point. Be positive, be empathetic to the other, be giving, be graceful and compassionate, be all of those lovely words that seemingly have nothing to do with what most of us really feel deep inside, through no fault of our own. How can we feel compassionate when we feel shitty about ourselves? How can we be giving when we feel that all everyone does with us is take and take? Some of us cannot even stand to be around positive people: "I hate people who constantly smile; they rub me the wrong way. Their smile feels fake to me / I feel like slapping them down." When we are feeling badly, and we feel badly much of the time (for an endless variety of reasons), we don't want to help anyone else, we don't want to let anyone take our place on the road or on the line for the supermarket / postal office / or in the various halls of bureaucracy. We don't want to listen to him and to his trouble (because we have enough of our own. "Let him handle his own baggage.") Generally, we are *far more irritable than we would like to be and far less patient than we would like to be.* It is no great prize to wade in the pool of negativity. To make it easier and more pleasant to handle ourselves in daily life, we *suppress the pain and/or ignore it and/or put on our happy masks and/or swallow pills to dull the aches of our body or the depression of our souls and pray for better days or to win the lottery. We survive.* Our survival instinct is certainly satisfied by this.

## *The soul as the mediator in the trilogy*

Yes, we are complex creatures. We are very complex creatures and, as we see, filled with inner conflicts. It is no wonder that we suffer so much. So how does this complex body-soul-spirit operation work?

| **Body** | **Soul** | **Spirit** |
|---|---|---|
| Temporal | Temporal | Eternal |
| **Body** | **Soul** | **Spirit** |
| Physical | Metaphysical | Metaphysical |

As we can see, two of our parts are temporal and one is eternal. There are also two parts that are metaphysical (they cannot be touched, seen and measured) and a single part that is physical-material. It is our soul that is both temporal (like our body) and metaphysical (like our spirit). It therefore has a super-important role as the mediating link between the temporal and the eternal and the physical and the metaphysical. In other words, our soul, through the varied and massive emotional and consciousness spectrum, actually mediates and provides a bridge between our body and the spirit and between the temporal and the eternal.

But why do we even need a bridge and a mediator? Because unlike the situation with the Waze application (to return to that analogy) which we spoke of earlier, where an electronic narrator provides semi-melodious instructions about "turning right in a few meters" and all that we are required to do is listen to the instructions and carry them out, we cannot hear the spirit in such a clear or obvious way. Aside from the basic fact that most of us are not aware of the spirit within us, there are other reasons that we cannot hear its voice: It is a "still, small voice" and it cannot penetrate the cacophonic background noise of our overloaded brain. It is easy to miss. So what does the spirit do? How does the eternal-wise part of us that desires our supernal good still reach our consciousness without speaking to us with words?

Thanks to its great intelligence and wisdom, the spirit has *various ways of expressing itself: It speaks to us through our feelings and sensations, through events that occur in our external reality, through dreams, through pain and diseases, through intuition, through gut feelings, through inspiring ideas that "suddenly" appear in our minds and through powerful epiphanies of the heart that sidetrack ordinary rationality.*

## So what do I feel or experience?

Let us start with our emotions and sensations. They are among the most important components of our essence and hence it is extremely important to be aware of them. What do we truly feel? When? With whom? Where? Moreover, why do we even feel that way? Our emotions oscillate on a scale ranging from the airy, joyful emotions of happiness, courage, confidence, serenity, belonging, acceptance, satisfaction, faith, compassion, caring, spontaneity and generosity to the harsher, more challenging, emotions of sadness, fear, disgust, shame, self-pity, anger, exhaustion, helplessness, boredom, arrogance, pain or indecision. Our sensations, which have an actual physical-sensory expression, have a wide-ranging scale ranging from sensations that are pleasant to the body, such as glee, relief, excitement, lightness, freshness, thrill, passion, desire, openness or wonderment to unpleasant sensations, such as confusion, panic, surprise, suffocation, isolation, nervousness, wrath, shakiness, vertigo, befuddlement, shock or cramps. *When we feel or experience feelings and sensations that we find pleasant, that is a sign that we are right where we are supposed to be at that given moment.* It could be that the rightness of the situation, event, meeting or location could change in a minute, a week, a month or a year, but for this specific moment, this situation, event, encounter or location is exactly right for us for the simple reason that it makes us feel good. The good feeling, you see, is the sign. *On the other hand, if we feel or experience unpleasant feelings or sensations, there is a story behind that negative experience as well.* That story could be something or someone that we are aware of or something which we are unaware of. But be sure, there is a reason to why we respond as we do since the spirit, body and soul are collaborating here. *The unpleasant feelings and sensations we feel and experience have two roles. The first is to indicate to us that we must choose between two options: To treat the situation and act in order to change it or to walk away. The second role of these unpleasant sensations and feelings is to shine a light onto our inner self.* This light reveals aspects of our soul that require attention, showing us where we should treat ourselves. For the most part, these aspects of our soul that are expressed in our fear, anger and pain derive from the personal biography of every one of us.

I will provide a few examples to illustrate this point:

We meet a specific person under personal (friend, significant other, family member) or professional (boss, colleague, client, mentor) circumstances and we feel happy and carefree with him. He makes us feel good about ourselves. A day or a week or a month or a year later that man betrays us or deeply hurts us. What does that mean? That we never should have met him in the first place? That it is a shame that that terrible man entered our life? Not at all. The first role of the unpleasant feelings and sensations is to direct us to the choice we must make -- do we choose to deal with the situation by having harsh words with this harmful individual, do we take some other remedial action (reporting, filing a complaint, getting professional help) or do we choose to walk away by having nothing more to do with this individual and getting him out of our lives? The second role of these unpleasant feelings and sensations is, as aforementioned, to shine a light on our inner selves. In this example, the injury itself is the turning point in our lives. The injury is an opportunity for self-reflection, for identifying, recalling and cleansing the injured aspect within us by recognizing it, clearing the associated emotional load associated to it and hence making a change -- growing and undergoing personal development thanks to the "offensive asshole" who hurt us. That is, in fact, our "lofty benefit" -- the beneficial development which grows from the evil thing which was done to us.

A certain individual can trigger a feeling of suffocation and nervousness every time we are near him. A certain perfume used by an individual can trigger disgust or cramps every time we smell it. A certain repetitive situation in our lives always irritates us or makes us feel helpless (constant criticism by a parent, disrespect or lack of common courtesy by a neighbor or associate, arrogance by a workplace colleague or verbal abuse by a relative). A certain place where we frequently go or pass by causes us to feel confusion or isolation. A certain food which truly disgusts us makes us shake every time we even think of it. There are infinite emotions and sensations which we experience during our everyday lives and the negative ones tell us a very detailed story.

How can we know who, in fact, is telling us this story? How do we know who it is that directs us, whether it is our eternal spirit or our temporal soul? The truth is that most of us will find it next to impossible to distinguish between the spirit and the soul because the *soul is, in fact, no more than a reflection of the spirit* and of the things that that spirit is here to experience, learn, express and create through our lives in this dense material universe. *The soul is the executive arm of the spirit*, that very same coach driver from the aforementioned analogy of the coach and the hidden passenger and they are interwoven with one another. Since the eternal spirit whispers and the temporal soul is drowning in an ocean of (mostly negative) thoughts, we may not know which of us is truly telling us the story right now. However, the bottom line is that *as far as our lives are concerned, it doesn't really matter which one of them is trying to reach our conscious mind through our unpleasant emotions and sensations, so long as we listen to the story they tell us* and act accordingly so that we might return to the positive emotions and sensations and to the place that is right for us and for our development.

## *What is actually happening to me here?*

Let us consider another way in which the wise and intelligent spirit, which is an inseparable part of us, speaks to us. It does so by promoting certain situations and events in our external reality. There are immediately beneficial situations such as being promoted at work, being accepted to the job of our dreams or a prestigious university, falling in love, getting married, a pregnancy and / or a birth, a pleasant and refreshing vacation, achieving our goals, fulfilling an old dream, moving to our dream house and so on. Beneficial situations, by their very nature, make us feel good, which is excellent and helpful for us. On the other hand, there are many unpleasant situations that lead us to feel and experience negative and even painful emotions and sensations. This *is where the story is. This is guidance. This is shining a light on the dark places and, above all else, this is an opportunity to change and grow.* When we are fired from our job, when we experience betrayal by a friend or significant other, when we experience divorce, when we experience humiliation, when we experience violence directed at our person, when we experience the death of a loved one or when we ourselves have a brush with death through a car accident, we are slapped by reality and, for a moment, we stop to reflect. That is simply the way we are. *We only leave the routine and our comfort zone under extreme conditions. We only take a break from our crazy rat race under extreme conditions. We only wake up from our sleepwalker existence under extreme conditions.* The shock and / or the pain leads us to shut ourselves off from the outside world and withdraw within because we feel like shit and because our social switch is turned off and we have no desire to see people. Therefore, we silence our engines for a moment. In the relative silence it is easier to hear the small still voice of the spirit. In this relative quiet it is easier to check up on ourselves. In this relative quiet it is possible to examine, truly examine, the circumstances of our lives. In this silence we can ask the questions which will direct us on the path to growth and perhaps even hear the answers that the spirit whispers in our direction when the time is right. In the relative silence we discover the courage to change course -- indeed, sometimes the situation forces us to change and recalibrate our bearings to the destination that is right for us on all levels -- physical, mental-emotional spiritual and energetic.

## Ouch, that hurts

Pain and disease are another version of extreme situations (ranging between flu and a cramp to cancer or paralysis). Here, too, there is a story, guidance, a shining of the light like a laser pointer into the inner dark and a chance for change and development. Here, too, there is an attempt to signal us to pull over for a moment and to begin to notice our neglected aspects because pain or diseases are physiological expressions of emotional-mental distress. A disease or a pain speaks to us about the untold tale of our soul. They hint to us (through their location in the body, their timing and their nature) that there is something we forgot about or suppressed in order to protect ourselves and that that something, that trauma, that pain-fear-anger is remerging back up to the surface in the shape of the illness and / or the physiological pain. Why now? Because now we are now prepared to face them, treat them, acknowledge them, unload the associated emotional baggage and all the emotional waste associated with that event and pass through the curtain of pain so that we can finally let go of it and thereby enable the healing, both mental and physical, to take place.

If we successfully detach ourselves for a moment and ascend above the pain and above our perceptions and beliefs about the negative nature of the disease and our bewildered "Why the hell has this happened to us?" If we can *reach that spiritual perspective which can see far more than the current point in time and space,* (In other words, transform ourselves into the navigational application that can see beyond the current irritating traffic jam.) then we can, from that interface point with the spirit, *see our supreme good (which is so much more than our immediate good). From there we can see the incredible opportunity for change, for discarding whatever does not support the true needs of our body and soul. From there we can see how to develop ourselves and our capabilities. From there we can see how we can reconnect to ourselves, what we really want to happen, what we truly want to do, what we truly feel and what truly benefits us. We can summon the courage to demand it, see from that vantage point that yes, we really do deserve it, that we truly are worthy of all the good in the world.*

The spirit can guide us in the process of change -- in its own special and gentle way which we must, of course, study. It will indicate to us how to treat ourselves, whom to seek out for assistance, what method to use, what path to follow and what action to take. Why? Because it desires the same things we do. It is "invested in us" in all senses of the word, because *if we do not reach our destination, neither will it.*

## *"Wow, I had such a crazy dream!"*

Our intelligent and wise spirit can also transmit messages to us through our dreams. In the diverse range of situations, events, nightmares, people (living or dead), places and traumas that appear in our dreams, we can also find *messages, solutions and direction from the spirit for the situation that we face or suppress while we are awake and conscious.* We do not remember most of our dreams. We recall them vaguely or forget them minutes after waking up. There are, on the other hand, *dreams which will not leave us even in our waking moments, dreams that are so powerful that we can recall them even after a great deal of time, dreams that we recall in great detail.* There is a reason why those dreams will not let us be.

A few words regarding dreams: There have been many attempts throughout history to decipher and unlock their meaning and significance. Ancient cultures viewed dreams as messengers, bearers of wisdom and therefore attributed them to the gods. In the Old Testament as well, when Pharaoh called upon Joseph to interpret his dream, Joseph answered: "It is not in me; God will give Pharaoh a favorable answer."

(Genesis: 41:16) In other words, in contemporary parlance, he told him to get off his case and to take it to God as he was the only one who could interpret his dreams. The Swiss psychiatrist Carl Gustav Jung, (once a well-known student of Sigmund Freud who split with him over professional differences,) who studied dreams for many years, tended to agree with cultures we now call "primitive" and was convinced that the dream was a story with its own logic, rhythm and even purpose. Jung claimed that *dream consciousness represented a higher and more holistic consciousness than that held by the waking mind* (in contrast to the assumption that the dream consciousness was inferior to the waking consciousness). Freud, on the other hand, saw the dream as a casual result of suppression. Suppressed energies of various impulses and forbidden urges that were not expressed in everyday life and that required some sort of outlet. As far as he was concerned, our internal moral police officer simply let the inmates vent some steam through dreams. I will add that psychologists and brain scientists who deal with the biological- physiological aspect of the brain (which is scientifically proven and that can be observed and measured), do not really agree upon a single definition of the role of dreams. Since psychologists view dreams as mental, rather than biological phenomenon -- *the I (the metaphysical part) is the one dreaming rather than the brain (the grey physical part) and everything connected to the "I" cannot be truly tested or proven scientifically* such as, for example, random twitches in the neurons of the brain or the movements of the eyeball. To summarize this brief historical review, we can say that the perspective which led humanity to attribute dreams to the gods (a dream knows something about ourselves that we do not that is derived from some superior consciousness that is not part of our own soul) cannot be proven scientifically. Scientists also agree that in anything related to dreams, in spite of all of the recent discoveries, the unknown is greater than the known.

The information, messages, solutions or guidance that the spirit passes on to us through dreams is transmitted in a way that is very symbolic (and not necessarily direct) and very individual. For example, should a certain model of a car, in a certain color, appear in our dream, that car might have a very different meaning for us (progression on our path) than its meaning to another dreamer (luxury, affluence, a vacation…). Even the color of the car can be highly significant for us and have no significance or a completely different significance, to another dreamer. The meanings of items, places, events or people who appear in our dreams are all related to the personal biography of each one of us, to our system of beliefs and to the conclusions that we have derived from the events we experienced in life. Perhaps we have a history with the item which appeared in our dream and that will be where the hint to solve the puzzle we face will come from. A dream of waves breaking upon the cliffs might be a symbol of our fear of crashing, a symbol of the end of a long journey, a symbol of power or a symbol for a type of slow erosion. A man we know who appears in our dream may symbolize heroism, foolishness, love, cowardliness or generosity, depending on what we know or think we know about this person. It all depends on what the symbol means to us.

To summarize the issue of dreams as a means of transmitting information from the spirit: We cannot really know for certain who is the party responsible for a specific message we receive in a dream. Is it an aspect of the temporal soul or of the eternal and wise spirit? If this is *information which will not leave us in peace, an image which remains sharp and clear in our mind or an idea which will not let us be, it certainly has a role in assisting us to reach our destination.* It is worthwhile to be a bit more proactive and to raise a question before you go to sleep. Oftentimes, answers will arrive in your dreams and they can surprise you. Try it. There is nothing to lose, just to gain.

**Carl Jung:**

> *"Within each of us exists another entity of which we are unaware. It speaks to us through our dreams and leads us to understand that it is completely different from what we perceive ourselves to be."*

## *"This somehow feels right..."*

We have reached the final way in which the eternal and wise spirit speaks to us. In my opinion, this is also the most interesting, exciting and tantalizing way, even if it is the vaguest and the least "scientific" of all of the aforementioned channels of communications. As far as I am concerned, it is also underappreciated in our modern life. *This path includes our gut feelings, our intuitions, our inspirations and the knowledge of our heart.*

*Who among us has never had moments in life in which he acted on a hunch?* A hunch which led us to walk in a path which was different than what we had planned (whether geographically or strategically), a hunch which led us to trust someone although we didn't know him well enough or a feeling which led us to choose something or someone who we never would have selected in an "ordinary" situation?

*Who among us never had a moment in life when he acted on intuition (the twin sister of the hunch)?* That silent knowledge which enabled us to know that someone was lying to us through his earnest expression, that he was sad in spite of his smile, whether he truly liked us, or, even in more extreme occasions, when the doctor told us that the medical examinations were sound but we still knew that there was "something wrong" (putting aside for the moment the poor hypochondriacs who are sure their entire lives that there is "something wrong").

*Who among us never had inspiring ideas that "suddenly" appeared in our head?* Grand ideas or solutions to various problems that appeared in our mind "out of nowhere," in the middle of washing dishes, taking a shower, weeding the garden, staring at the screen, daydreaming or any situation which allows us a modicum of relaxation or release (a basic systemic requirement for the appearance of those ideas)? Some of the greatest inventors and scientists, whose default state was rational, organized and logical thinking, reached insights, discoveries, inventions and scientific theories which changed the world by listening to their intuition. Or else their ideas appeared in their dreams or suddenly appeared in their mind while they were enjoying a few moments of "temporary system shutdown" (light rest, staring at nothing, reflection). Famous examples are Newton who, when watching an apple fall from a tree, came up with the basic principles of gravity and Archimedes, who, while taking a soak in bath, suddenly understood (Eureka!) the basis of the displacement principle. In any event, the *paradox of scientific breakthroughs (the greatest discoveries in science were not discovered in preplanned and organized scientific process)* is an excellent example of this means in which the spirit transmits messages to us.

*Who among us has not had powerful epiphanies of the heart that bypassed every rational argument or knowledge?* Epiphanies whose truth touched us so deeply even though they contradicted what we or those near us thought or believed beforehand? Epiphanies which led us to make odd and even seemingly delusional choices *but which we knew were the right choices for us* and never had any need to muck about or questions ourselves? Epiphanies such as "I knew she would be my wife the first time I met her." "I just knew I had to leave this profession." "I knew I had to go study special education / acting / art even though my parents opposed this and wanted me to study medicine / law / accounting / any other profession with money in it." "I knew it was right for me to live in this state on the other side of the world." "I knew he was the right mentor / partner for me." "I knew I had to write this book" or "I always knew that that was what I was meant to do in the world." Almost all of us have had these epiphanies. Whether we do anything with them or not is a completely different question and one we will discuss later on.

To summarize this part, yes, our spirit is creative and diverse and has infinite paths of reaching us, guiding us, helping us and marking the path leading to our supreme benefit. When we are aware of the existence of the spirit ("Oh, so we have this part within us in addition to all the other clutter? Well, that's good to know.") and to the sophisticated and sometimes over clever ways it has of "speaking" to us (dreams / signifying events / challenging emotions / inner feelings / diseases and other treats), then collaboration between the three parts ensues. This leads to bidirectional attentiveness and communication and we can then begin to *perceive reality differently and begin to identify the mechanisms which inhibit and encourage our growth. Then, and only then, can we begin to accept the circumstances of life, particularly the difficult ones, in spite of the pain and difficulties they hold because we finally understand that some hidden message or lesson has been designed to take us to the next step of our development.* This is true whether it is truly a life changing event such as being fired or whether it is every day events such as someone cutting into the line at the supermarket, a colleague lying baldly to our face, unsupportive spouses, cheeky offspring, relatives who do not invite us to a family event, friends who badmouth us or a boss who ignores our needs.

## From spirit to spirituality in practice

If we take an additional step and become aware of this part within us, of this eternal and wise spirit, then we fulfill the essence of the word spirituality. We will dwell on this point for a moment if only because the word "spirituality" has become almost a curse word to certain people (just like the word "God"). And yet, it is but a word, not the thing itself -- like the difference between saying, "I fell in love" and actually feeling the thing itself and falling in love with someone. A vast chasm separates the two. This word "spirituality" (again, just like the word "God"), generates a great deal of antagonism and bears on its shoulders so many resentful residues and sacks of emotional detritus (for many different reasons), that it is worthwhile to take a moment to clarify what "being spiritual" actually means. Once we agree on the definition, we can be sure that we are synchronized and actually talking about the same thing.

*Being spiritual means living life in harmony between our three parts -- body, soul and spirit. In other words, to maintain a tri-directional data transfer both from the eternal to the temporal and from the metaphysical to the physical and back.* Being spiritual means living daily life *out of a desire to maintain this communication, out of a desire to receive guidance, out of a desire to find the signs, hear the spiritual entities that offer us guidance, identify the supportive probabilities and the opportunities as they emerge in the reality of our lives and not later, in retrospect.* That is how we can become more focused, proactive and initiating rather than wrapped up in confused, passive, reactive, helpless and negative victim-like emotions most of us feel in our daily life.

It is important that we differentiate between two identical and seemingly overlapping concepts that will assist us in the next chapter to further fine-tune the definition of spirituality and therefore make our work with the trilogy system more precise and maximize the benefit we will derive from it. These concepts are spiritual awareness and spiritual development. *Spiritual awareness is awareness of aspects beyond those that are apparent, awareness of everything beyond what our five senses perceive, through which we perceive and experience the world.* Remember the clinical death fellows we spoke of earlier? Those who died and came back to life? Those people have spiritual awareness -- they are aware of the world beyond the physical because they saw it and experienced it -- so they know it is there. No one and no argument in the world can take that experience or knowledge that an afterlife actually exists. Does this make them spiritual? Does this mean they live their lives with constant conscious communication between their three parts? Does this mean they seek to live their lives from within that essential unity / compassion / love which they met in their short trip in the world beyond? Not necessarily. Not at all. Take these people we define as spiritual or "new agers," "hippies." etc. (or any other disparaging definition we stick to anyone wearing robes, growing dreadlocks and pinning feathers in their hair), who read books about clinical death experiences / the afterlife / and various faiths and religions, who go to workshops where they listen to channeled angels and extra-dimensional beings. Does all that mean they are spiritual in their actions? Does any of that mean they live their lives with conscious communication between their three parts? No, not necessarily. Not at all. There is a massive difference between knowing something and implementing this knowledge in practice as all the people who know exactly what the right food for them is or what the ideal diet for their body is and yet find themselves eating empty carbs and sugars or processed foods filled with preservatives. This is the painful and challenging difference between knowing something and implementing it, the difference between knowledge and wisdom -- implementation in practice. By the way, just so we do not feel too badly about ourselves, I will note that some of the greatest teachers and mentors fail in this test, including some spiritual mentors, including men and women of the cloth. They teach one thing and act in contradiction to their own teachings. They teach us to show empathy and compassion and treat their own family or employees badly. They teach self-love and yet they abuse themselves (drugs / alcohol / gambling / abusive relationships…). They teach, *"Love your neighbor as yourself"* and display racism towards those who are different. No one is impervious to the test of implementation, if only because we are all human.

The second concept which is important to precisely define before we proceed onwards is that of "spiritual development." When a man develops spiritually, in reality, in practice, he develops in two parallel channels: He develops emotionally and develops his consciousness. On the emotional level, he acknowledges and learns additional aspects of the soul, mostly the deepest and least sexy, which are expressed in awareness of what we feel, what we fear, what we are ashamed of, what hurts us, what disturbs our calm and what makes us angry. *On the conscious level*, this is, in fact, *self-awareness* that is expressed by awareness to why and how we act the way we do, why we react as we do in a conversation with parents / friends / spouses / children and why we think damaging thoughts about ourselves.

So if we bring the question "Who is a spiritual individual?" down to basics, it would seem to be *an individual who implements the spiritual knowledge in the reality of his own life* (for example, in an effort to implement, "Love thy neighbor as thy love thyself," to love ourselves and others; for example to attempt to implement "Turn from evil and do good," on ourselves and others, or for example, to attempt to implement, "Keep your tongue from evil and your lips from deceit," to do your best not to gossip, deceive or lie) *and so does a man who is connected to himself, who knows himself and the myriad layers of his soul, who is aware of his thoughts, desires, needs and behavior and who acts out of that knowledge.* When we are present in that connected place, we are actually connected to our own essence, connected also to the spirit within us. We listen to and are attentive to it, to ourselves and therefore meet the definition of spirituality. It is at that point that we can be defined as a spiritual people. Does that mean that our lives are perfect, calm and free of strife? Not at all. The spiritual path is not one that is free of barriers, challenges or even nerves and fears but it certainly enables us to understand the higher reasons for their occurrence and to see them as means of development and hence to control our reactions and select the optimal path for us at those points in time.

And yet, in spite of all that has been said so far, 90% of the time we are consciously aware and recall only the two "celebrities,"-- our body and our soul. Only rarely do we turn our thoughts to "the new kid on the block," that eternal part within us that always was and always will be, that nearly hidden part. In order to increase the part that the spirit plays in our everyday life, we must remember and remind ourselves that it exists, remember and remind ourselves to listen to it, remember and remind ourselves of the many manifest advantages imbued in being attentive to the knowledge that it is transmitting to us. How do we remind ourselves? This is a process that is much like training in a gym, driving or learning how to play an instrument. You must repeat, practice and train repeatedly, time after time, and eventually, it is imbued in the system. Eventually, the neural pathways in the mind, which make an action quicker and even automatic, thicken. Eventually the habit is seared into the subconscious and then you no longer need to think of the actions -- you just do them. Eventually, you remember that the spirit is there, within us, half of the time, at best.

## Ancient wisdom in the test of time

Just so that we are all synchronized, all of the aforementioned regarding the three parts of man is not new. On the contrary, this is very ancient information which was prevalent among the educated and priestly classes of the ancient world -- in Egypt, in Greece, in Tibet, in China, in India, among the native North American nations, the Toltecs in Mexico[3], the Mayans of Central America, mystical Judaism (The Kabballah -- the code breaking of the occult), the Islamic Sufis and the teachings of Jesus and Buddha as well. *They all spoke the same eternal truth, coloring it with different hues* that fit the various cultures, customs, times and places and of course the personal idiosyncrasies of each philosopher, teacher, priest or shaman. In other words, *over the years, this same wisdom, this same intelligence, wore different masks.*

So, if the entire world was aware of this spiritual truth, how could we, in our supposedly educated and enlightened western society, remain almost completely unaware of any of this? By "we" I mean the common people, the masses.

The first reason is linked to the fact *that this knowledge was never truly the province of everyone. It was never shared with the masses* -- not in the ancient city-states and certainly not in the villages or the wild forests. Furthermore, unlike our experience today, the masses in the past were illiterate, uneducated and frightened (that is, after all, how they were ruled) and all they knew was what their rulers told them (whether through heralds in the city square or by the nightly campfire). That was the way things were for thousands of years, from the dawn of civilization to the very recent past. Only in the past few generations, in the modern era, has this knowledge trickled and spread slowly around the globe, mostly thanks to the internet, allowing more and more of the "masses" to be exposed to it. Just as you are being exposed to

---

3      See "The Four Agreements" by Miguel Ruiz.

it in this book, right now.

The second reason is associated with the fact that over the years a gradual *separation* has developed. At first, there was merely a *separation from the spirit,* a focus on what was perceived by the five senses. Over time, we have arrived at a situation where science either denies or at best *ignores our soul as well and the effect of our beliefs and our emotions on our reality.* We can easily see this in everything that is related to modern medicine that resolves aches and pains by treating solely the human body (and the biological-physiological-biochemical processes within it) while blatantly ignoring the various aspects of the soul, both apparent and hidden, that are linked to that disease or pain and / or caused them. *The irony is that the same renowned science which we worship (and need) has already "scientifically" proved, on more than one occasion, that both our consciousness and our emotions effect solid matter and transform it.* (We will expand on this in the third part of the trilogy, in the prelude to "Why did we create this situation?")

The third reason is linked to the fact that we, in modern western society based on modern technology, are rather *arrogant.* We think *we know everything,* particularly given that over the past twenty years, with the entry of Google into our lives (and all the crazy bits of knowledge it brings with it) *and we tend to look down at the wisdom of the past.* After all, it is outdated and anachronistic. How can it be anything else when it comes to us from a period where no science existed and there was not much knowledge about the universe we live in (or even knowledge about what occurred beyond the small village where people were born, lived and died). There was no electricity and no global communication network? What could those old fogies possibly know about life, anyway? Whatever they might have known in ancient times was relevant to those times and is irrelevant to the modern era, just as analog-based devices are irrelevant to the intensive, rapid, interlinked and smart digital age. We place innovation and the latest upgrades on a pedestal and by that same measure dismiss all ancient knowledge or at least treat it like extinct dinosaurs. It was once and it is gone now. Farewell.

What do we forget along the way? We forget that thousands of years ago, even if there was no electricity-television-communication network and even if there was no clear knowledge of the cosmos, the stars or the molecular structure of a living cell, *people, ignorant as they might have been, were just as human as you and I,and dealt with the joys, challenges, pains and fears of life just as we do*. There were annoying relatives we did not feel like seeing and there were friends who did not always support. There were economic difficulties, there was love, there was betrayal, there was grief, there was heartbreak and there was heartbreak at the death of loved ones. There were triumphs and achievements, there was theft, there was fornication, there was laughter and there were diseases and accidents that ended life all too soon. Moreover, there was even wine to make the heart of man merry. Our ancestors felt the entire emotional spectrum we do and nothing in that regard has changed in this day and age -- even if the present is more materially comfortable than the past (we have toilets, air conditioners and flowing water) -- even if we have no fear of starvation (but are often starved emotionally) and even if all of the enormous knowledge the world has to offer is only a single mouse click away.

Doesn't it seem to you worthwhile to make use of the enormous knowledge accumulated at no small investment of blood, sweat and tears throughout all of human history and from all corners of the earth? If that same eternal truth (even if decked in various costumes and multi-colored hues) tells us that we are made up of three parts -- body, soul and spirit -- and that communication and connection between the three will help us grow, develop and open us up -- or at least make our life a bit easier, isn't it worth taking a moment to stop and listen? If that faith teaches us that so long as we are severed from our spirit, we will not be truly whole and that "something will always be missing" regardless of how many assets we acquire, isn't it worth it to pull over and try to figure out how regaining our connection with our spirit can improve our everyday life? Even if we do need to figure out how to "upgrade" this ancient wisdom to the 3$^{rd}$ millennium, isn't it worth it?

## Summary of part 1-- the three parts of man

- Man is made up of three parts: The temporal body, the temporal soul and the eternal spirit.

- The perspective of the spirit: Eternal and immortal, a high vantage point that looks upon life from a bird's eye view, is concerned with the lessons our life is supposed to teach us. It acts from an existence of cosmic, non-linear, interdependent time where everything occurs simultaneously and no space-time limitations exist.

- The spirit is essentially a mixture of supreme grace and a universal harmony of compassion, love, calm, serenity, acceptance and a superior intellect that enables near automatic understanding of "Why things are as they are."

- If we compare the spirit to the Waze navigation application, it has all of the data regarding all of the possible routes we might take and it knows the destination – where each of them leads. It does not interfere with our choices and merely offers us the optimal alternative given its analysis of all of the data.

- The spirit speaks in a small, still voice and it is difficult for us to hear it in this noisy and chaotic world, particularly given our thick, emotional defenses.

- The spirit is creative and varied in its approaches: It has an infinite number of paths in which it can reach us and mark the way leading to our supreme good.

- It speaks to us through our feelings and sensations (shining a light on the inner dark), through manipulating situations in our external reality (opportunities for change and development), through dreams (guidance and messages that are transmitted through individualized symbolism), through pains and diseases (opportunities to discard that which does not support the body and the soul), through hunches and intuitions (which motivate us to action even in the absence of a sufficient logical explanation), through inspiring ideas which "suddenly" appear in our head (in moments of "temporary shutdown" such as light rest, staring at the air, reflection, serenity or relaxation) and through powerful epiphanies of the heart (which bypass all sense and logic).

- Awareness of the spirit's sophisticated style of "speech" leads to recognition of our growth-delaying and growth-promoting mechanisms and to the acceptance of the circumstances of life through the understanding that they are imbued with a lesson which is meant to take us to the next step of our development.

- A spiritual man manages an ongoing and tri-directional communication between body, soul and spirit out of a desire to receive guidance, find the signs of this guidance, be exposed to the superior intellect of the spirit and to identify supportive probabilities and opportunities as they arise in his life.

- A man who develops spiritually develops both emotionally and in his consciousness while implementing the spiritual knowledge in the reality of his life and getting to know himself in all of the various layers of his soul.

# The Three Premises

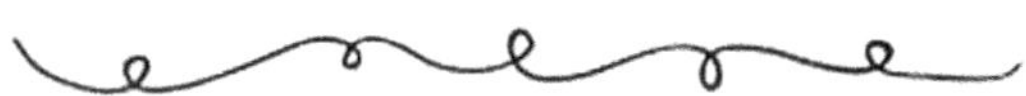

*Opportunities show up in disguise*

*Self-compassion, not berating oneself*

*Every setback is an opportunity
for growth*

In this part, we will go over the three premises that serve as a starting point to the inner exploration that we will perform when we ask ourselves the three questions of the trilogy method. These three premises are:

1. **Opportunities show up in disguise**
2. **Self-compassion, not berating oneself**
3. **Every setback is an opportunity for growth**

# 1 Opportunities Show Up in Disguise

*Who asked for an opportunity and didn't receive it?*

Someone wise once said that the definition of luck is "opportunity meets readiness." The truth is that all of us run into opportunities throughout our lives. The question is: What do we do with them? Are we prepared for them? Do we even recognize them? Are we prepared for the price we must pay in order to fulfill the opportunity that comes our way? Are we prepared to change what must be changed in order to fulfill it? Can we accept it? Do we even believe that we are worthy of this opportunity? Does this opportunity frighten us to the very marrow of our bones and even paralyze us and prevent us from responding to the appearance of opportunity?

Some of the opportunities which appear in our lives are essentially positive -- things we have yearned for, prayed for, desired and even intrigued and fantasized about (the right man, a job interview in the right place, the right spouse, the right home, the right financing, the right mentor, the right outfit, the right message...). Unfortunately, reality tends to mainly present us with opportunities that are difficulties or challenges that force us to leave our comfort zone --

something we do not always want to do. Generally speaking, we prefer not to move or change things. Perhaps we prefer not to admit it *but most of us prefer the known and familiar difficulties we know over an unfamiliar opportunity -- even if it has the potential to lead us to better places.* Why is this, you might ask? Why would we prefer to give up an opportunity for something better? It makes no sense, does it? Well, other than the fact that where strong emotions are involved (particularly negative emotions), mind and logic do not necessarily take center stage. *There are a few other reasons such as a preference to clinging to the known, fear of the unknown, our habits having the upper hand in most situations and, above all else, non-recognition of opportunities.*

I will illustrate this tendency to cling to the familiar and fear of the unknown with a rather extreme example which will nonetheless get the point across. Let us say that one day we discover or become aware of the fact that we have been wallowing in a pool of literal shit, that it stinks and that we are sticky, dirty and wet (go wild with any other repugnant association you can think of). We do not really know how to get out of this mucky pool, we see no positive horizon in sight and perhaps we are close to drowning in the pool. Then, one day, an opportunity to escape arises -- an unknown hand is extended to us and offers to pull us out. The logical thing to do is, of course, bless our good fortune and grab on to that hand, right? Nonetheless, most of us will not do that. Why? Because we rationalize that yes, we are wallowing in shit but we are used to this shit, know it and its boundaries like the palm of our hand, know where everything is and know everyone who is stuck in this shit with us. Sure, it is a bit stinky but it is also nice and warm and outside it is cold, cloudy and perhaps even stormy, and whose hand is it anyway? Who knows who he is or what his interests are? Perhaps he only wants to pull us out in order to harm us? Besides, who promised us that the outside world is any better? Who knows, maybe it is worse out there and then we will lose our place here in the shit pool and end up with nothing? What if our hand slips as we try to pull ourselves out and we drown? Good God, this is all far too terrifying, better not to even think about it (and here the avoidance / suppression / paralysis mechanism kicks in or a good old panic attack if all else fails).

Well, perhaps this example seems slightly ridiculous to us but this is in fact how we act. Why? Because we hate living in uncertainty. It unsettles us, stresses us out, threatens us and frightens us. We will do everything to avoid uncertainty since, under such conditions, we are not in control and that is something we simply cannot permit ourselves, it drives us nuts. Since we do not want to be in this place of uncertainty, we would rather cling to what is known and familiar, which is wherever we are now -- even if that is wallowing in the same old pool of shit.

Let us adapt this extreme example to our more familiar daily lives. The clinging to the known and the familiar and the hatred of uncertainty that characterize us means that our personal pool of shit can be many things. It can be remaining in an unsatisfying / non rewarding job, sticking to a tiring / hated/ unfulfilling boring profession, remaining friends with people that are not interesting / not supportive / irrelevant, staying under an oppressive / harassing / marionette boss, staying with a violent / unsupportive / inappropriate / humiliating spouse, continuing to study / specialize in a field we hate / are tired of instead of learning something new / something we always dreamed about in our heart of hearts or living in the same environment / city / village even though it isn't good for us there and we fantasize about life in another environment that will match our true needs. It even includes clinging to various harmful addictions such as smoking / alcohol / drugs / overeating or devouring sweets. After all, we know just what will happen and what we will feel once we drink, eat or puff on that cigarette or joint (in the short term we will enjoy the taste, the buzz, the calm and the fun feeling). This knowledge comforts us, even though the act harms us and is damaging to us in the long term.

## It is all about neural pathways in our brain

*The other reason most of us prefer the difficulties we know and are familiar with over unfamiliar opportunities is related to the triumph of our habits.* The habits I am referring to are both bodily and behavioral and are expressed in thought, word and deed. This is where we can find a quantum of solace -- there is a clear physiological-neurological reason for the strength of our habits that explains why it is so hard for us to change them. *That reason is related to the formation of neurological pathways in our brain.* What does that mean? Every action / thought / emotion that we have is expressed in neural activity in our brain (electric pulses that are fired by our neural cell.

The brain is made up of trillions of such neural cells).

Whenever we repeat a given behavior or activity time after time and pulses are fired from the specific neural cells associated with this activity / behavior, neural pathways are formed in the brain which will, in time, grow and therefore also make our actions faster and more automatic. As time goes by and as this action is repeated, these tiny pathways grow to become a type of a "highway." Then we do not even need to think about the action. It happens on its own. It is easy to understand this basic brain activity when we think about studying a new skill like driving or playing an instrument. At first, these activities seem hard to us. They feel unnatural, clumsy, confusing and we need to constantly think and correct mistakes in their performance, all with a great deal of frustration.

Over time, with sufficient training and persistence, just like weight training when we try to build up our muscle mass, these new skills become easy, enjoyable, require very little thought and our muscles move to a semi-automatic mode. It doesn't matter whether the action is playing an instrument, driving or any other type of activity. The longer we persist and train at it and the more we repeat the action, the electric pulses fired from those neuronal cells associated with these actions are added to the "musical instrument path" or the "driving path." Therefore, these neural pathways grow and become stronger and faster and with time and repetitiveness of the action, they become sort of fast and wide highways that bring you to your destination very rapidly compared to less-used, narrower, roads. On the physiological level, it has been scientifically proven that the structure and function of our brain constantly change in accordance with what we do, think or speak, thanks to our neuroplasticity[4].

The explanation and example provided here for learning how to drive or play a musical instrument are equally valid for behaviors and responses. If we are in the habit of being judgmental or negative, if we tend to see the glass half empty, if we react impulsively without thinking things through, if we always think of the worst thing that can happen in any situation, if we do not trust people, if we complain or blow off steam every time we go through something, the neural paths associated with those habits will thicken. Depressing? Not when you consider that if get into the habit of being optimistic, if we always look at the glass half full, if we make a habit of listening to people and helping them, then those positive thoughts, responses and behaviors and their continuous repetitions will thicken the neural pathways associated with

---

4     You can find simple, easy to understand, explanations for those of us who are not brain surgeons from the field of neuroscience in the fascinating book "The Brain that Changes Itself" by Norman Doidge. This book will help you understand more deeply why it is so hard for you to change your habits but will also prove to you that they can be changed and, in fact, that everything can be changed! You can read there about the congenitally blind who have learned how to see, deaf people who learned how to hear, people with brain damage who were pronounced "incurable" who were completely rehabilitated and other traumas, obsessions and learning disorders that were completely cured. You will understand that nothing in our brain is permanent or unchangeable -- if you want to do something about it.

those positive behaviors or beliefs into highways, making the beliefs or behaviors semi-automatic and transforming what we define of our character and how we know ourselves.

Our character is made up of many habits: We are used to responding as we do, we are used to behaving as we do, we are used to thinking as we think and we are used to talking as we talk. We are so used to all of our old patterns that that is precisely why it is so hard for us to change them. It is far easier to take the well-traveled highway rather than blaze a new path in the wilderness, isn't it? It takes far less effort, even if science has proven that the structure of the brain can be changed and that nothing is permanent and unchangeable, not even the regulation of our genes,[5] it is still very difficult to do it in practice. It is very difficult to change something that we are used to since it requires mental force, dedication, perseverance, courage, a whole slew of other qualities we do not necessarily possess as well as the ability to rise up again after a fall. There are always falls on the path of changing something permanent and creating something new.

For example, if we try to bring optimistic thinking into our life, then the pessimistic thinking that we are used to and which we automatically draw upon in any given situation

---

5     Bruce Lipton: "Biology of Belief." Among other things, he demonstrates that stem cells grown with different types of mature cells differentiated, that is changed the epigenetics governing gene expression. There are numerous other examples of the expression and regulation of genes being changed by the environment (such as nutrition), including, **and this is very important**, human beliefs, thoughts and emotions.

is our highway and optimism is a new path we must create from nothing, for it does not yet exist. If we compare this to blazing a new path in the jungle, this will require a great deal of work -- chopping vegetation out of the way with a machete, uprooting stones, fallen logs and other obstacles off the path, filling potholes and leveling the surface. The conditions in which this backbreaking labor is performed are themselves difficult -- the jungle is hot, we are sweat drenched and there are annoying mosquitoes. It is all very exhausting and you need to work really hard until the new path is formed. And it needs to be traveled many times until it is comfortable and until it can bring us to our destination rapidly and with ease. Moreover, other people need to walk the path that we have blazed for it to slowly widen and become the highway it can be.

So can we train to become optimistic people even if we were pessimistic people for most of our lives? Can we train to become accepting of people as they are even if we were critical for most of our lives? Can we train ourselves to listen to what other people have to say even if we have grown used to dominating conversations over most of our lives? Can we train to learn to love ourselves even if we have hated ourselves for most of our lives? Can we work out and take care of our body even if we are used to neglecting and harming it? In theory, everything is possible. Through thought coupled with action, the brain can change its structure and function but it is hard, very hard, even though not impossible. It is difficult to blaze this new path in the jungle, this new habit or means of expression or behavior. It is far easier to do what we are used to doing, far easier to drive down the highway. It is natural for us and we do it on autopilot without thinking which is exactly why our habits usually have the better of us.

## Masks, and not just on Halloween...

*The final reason why most of us prefer the known difficulty over the unfamiliar opportunity is linked to the fact that we almost never recognize opportunity when we meet it since it is disguised and masked.* What is a mask? It is a type of illusion. We see one thing but it is actually something else and that something else lies under the mask and is hidden from view. Of course there are better disguises / masks and worse disguises / masks. There are different qualities and levels of credibility and there are different levels of connection and emotional engagement with the disguise (ranging from the man who is really excited by and lives the persona he adopts to the man who wanders around with a hangdog expression because "they made me dress up in this costume for the work party"). Still, as far as opportunities go, we usually trust the masks they don, just like a child believes in a good, high quality costume. A grownup, in contrast, immediately knows it for what it is and does not believe it or what it represents, not even for a single moment. He can enjoy it but he knows it isn't real because he sees beyond the immediately apparent.

Do all of our opportunities appear in disguise? No, but the more challenging ones certainly do. The opportunities we call positive are readily apparent and we recognize them straight out, whether they are economic, personal, professional or domestic. These include a promotion in our workplace or an opportunity for relocation to another state, being asked out on a date, being accepted to a prestigious institution of higher learning (for either our children or ourselves), a large inheritance, an offer of partnership in an interesting startup and so forth. We are aware that this is a great opportunity for us and respond with great joy and excitement. However, what happens when we face more challenging opportunities, ones that our autopilot categorizes as negative? This includes being laid off, a divorce, being rejected by an organization or a person, being cheated on, suffering from a disease, an accident, a fall and so forth? Well, when that happens, we are not excited to say the least and we certainly do not think that the event might lead us to a better place. We do not wonder whether we can learn something new from the event, grow stronger, meet new people, get better or get to know ourselves and our abilities better.

We cannot see all the options imbued in that opportunity because they are hidden, because they are disguised as something else and that disguise saddens, angers or frightens us or all three together. That is why the costume confuses us, just like the child who is scared when he sees a costume of an imp or a monster. The place where we strive to get to and which we can in fact reach, is to be that adult who can see through the costume, see it as what it is and therefore not truly believe in it and thereby see beneath it to its true nature.

*When we want something, the opportunity arrives in disguise.*

"True nature" means that beneath the opportunity lies our will, our true desire and it is it that we must explore, discover and thereby exploit the opportunity that has come knocking at our door. Why is investigation called for? Because there is a difference between what we think we want -- the apparent will -- and what we truly desire -- the hidden will. Indeed, in many cases they do not overlap in the least. Sometimes, it is hard for us to know what our true desires are, what we really want, because they are hidden beneath a sophisticated coating of the wills of others in our immediate environment (parents, spouses, children, friends, colleagues, family) and we find ourselves wanting what they told us that they want and / or what they told us is right for us. Our true desires can be hidden (or buried) -- even below a coating of environmental or cultural conditionings (about what is customary, accept-able, polite or expected) or beneath economic considerations, particularly existential-survival considerations that suppress any will that is not related to our daily struggle for survival. (For example, there is no point in discussing a desire to fulfill or self-actualize ourselves when there is a giant overdraft in the bank.) In other words, *if we summarize what we have said so far, we do not always recognize opportunities (because they appear in disguise)nor are we always aware of what we truly want with ourselves, with others or with life itself.*

Complicated? Confusing? This is the time to add another

layer to the bundle that is the human individual. In the first chapter, we spoke of the three parts of man -- body, spirit and soul. This is where we make the connection between our desires and these three parts. This is also where we dwell upon the significance of the temporal soul having certain desires (be they conscious or subconscious) that may not be identical or synchronized to those of the eternal spirit. In order to minimize the gap between the two and, in particular, the frustration caused by that gap, it is important to recognize and distinguish between the two types of desires -- those of the temporal soul and those of the eternal spirit. As we have seen in the first chapter, the spirit and the soul are distinct and separate from each other in nearly all parameters (perspective, essence, intelligence and creativity and the manner in which they transmit messages). It is therefore quite reasonable to conclude that their desires would also be different and distinct.

## *The desires of the temporal soul*

Let us start with the simpler, more familiar and therefore easier type of desire to understand -- the desires of the temporal soul. There are those desires of which we are more aware (mostly such material and physical desires such as making a living, shopping, a fit body, pampering vacations, relationships and children) and also desires of which we are not necessarily aware (more emotional desires, mostly the basic, even existential desires). These desires lurk below the surface of our mind, in its deeper layers. These include the need for a feeling of belonging (I want to be part of a family

/ a group / the gang), the need for love (I want to be loved / to love myself), the need for visibility (I want to be seen / to be treated, I am here!), the need for self-worth (I want to feel equal to others / to have value / to be worthy / to be valued by others), the need for expression (I want to be listened to / to be expressed / I also have what to say), the need for security (I want to know that I am protected, I want to feel safe, to have someone to rely on) and so forth.

At the level of the soul, if we want something, the opportunity will come. However, as we already mentioned, it comes in disguise and therefore we cannot always identify what is beneath its costume. For example, if we are somewhat cowardly people and we want to be more courageous in our lives, then, at some point, you can count on a roaring lion entering our lives. Why should such a scary and threatening thing enter our lives? Because this is our chance to be brave. The challenge that scares us most arrives so that we might have the opportunity to behave and respond differently, a chance to reprogram our autopilot, what we are used to doing. What are we used to doing when faced with such a threat? Scream in panic and flee or gather our courage and fight it? Probably fleeing hysterically because that is the most human thing to do. (There is no shame in wanting to stay alive. That is the instinct we all have in common.) However, if deep inside we desire a change and want to do things somewhat differently, an opportunity will arise that will include the potential for this change.

Yes, we can certainly say that these costumes are a tricky and confusing thing. That is why we generally believe the costume -- that is what we see on the surface, what is apparent. We barely perceive the opportunity disguised beneath it. And if we perceive it, we don't recognize it or recognize it -- only retroactively, after a long time has gone by. We are physically and emotionally separated from the thing itself which is why we recognized and understood exactly what was there, what the higher meaning of that event in our life was, how it affected us on the macro level and what paths it has led us on. Something similar happens when we ask a friend for advice and he, thanks to his emotional detachment from the events he did not personally experience, can recognize the opportunity and can therefore offer us good advice, soothe us or else direct us in a direction we would never have thought of on our own.

Before we transition to specific examples that will illustrate the sneakiness of the disguises and the confusion that they elicit (and these will be examples that have nothing to do with a roaring lion which few of us are likely to meet on a distant savannah), I will stress an important point: *Yes, the disguised nature of the opportunities we will come across, requires that we perform some hard, and not always attractive, internal work.* Indeed, we may not always be aware of the option of self-awareness (awareness of our thoughts, actions and behavior, the ability to look at ourselves from the outside).

*This will force us to investigate and explore what we truly desire.* What do our deeper layers truly want? Why has this opportunity come knocking at our door? What truth lies behind it? What is the true opportunity that the threatening / annoying / frightening / shocking / frustrating / painful costume is concealing from us? And yes, *a great deal of honesty and a pinch of courage are required here.* It is not always pleasant to look in the mirror and to face everything you see in it. It may be that it will show us aspects of ourselves which are not very complimentary, sides of our personality which we may try to conceal from the environment (and from ourselves in some cases). It may be that demons and shadows from the past will emerge, the kind of demons that we thought we had escaped, forgotten about, repressed, that we had shoved down into the basement and thrown away the key. Well, guess what? They are still there. They didn't go anywhere and in all of the years that have gone by they were only lying in wait, just waiting for the right opportunity to raise their heads, waiting for us to develop the emotional and mental maturity that would let us deal with them: To shine a light upon them and look them in the eye. To admit their existence, to accept them, to forgive them (perhaps even thank them) and then to let them go with love, to discharge the emotional waste and limiting systems of associated belief which they had stored within them all those years.

*The hard truth is that our demons have not really been sleeping away quietly all these years. They are the ghost in the machine that has been running so many of our "autopilot" re-sponses.* It is they which were partially responsible for why we respond as we respond to situations / people / events in our life. It is they which were responsible for why we feel as we feel in certain situations / with certain people / certain events in our life. It is they which were responsible for why we speak as we speak in certain situations / with certain people / at certain events in our life. We simply were not aware of this connection between ourselves and our demons, aware of this deeper layer within us which is exactly what we are beginning to do here, very slowly.

## *It only seems to be the opposite of what we want*

Here are a few specific examples that will illustrate the cunning and that same confusion that the disguises generate when seeking opportunities in the complex combination of the deeper and forgotten layers of our true self (referring solely to the desires of the soul). As we go over these examples, it is important to note that the event that occurs is seemingly the exact opposite of what we would wish but that this opposition is only on the surface -- below the mask lies the true significance of the event:

- We want to take a pampering, relaxing vacation but suffer from a traffic accident that grounds us in bed for a good long while.

- We want to move to a certain country but cannot get the required entry permit or work visa.

- We want and desire a promotion at work (believing that we are worthy, dedicated and doing a good job) and instead find ourselves fired.

- We want our family to pay us more attention and for someone to care about what we have to say and then find out they established a WhatsApp group that leaves us out.

- We want to increase the number of clients and instead trigger a wave of departing clients.

- We want to expand our business and find out that our partner has defrauded us and left us penniless.

- We want to start to invest more in our self-development, and our spouse informs us that he wants a divorce.

- We want to lose weight, we started a strict diet a week ago and suddenly there are a number of events and occasions in a row that drop our chances of sticking to our diet to zilch.

- We want to strengthen our faith and something "bad" happens that completely undermines it, raising many doubts about our universe and our place in it.

- We want to publish songs that we have written and receive deadly criticism from someone whose professional opinion we value highly.

- We want to start living a healthier life and find out that we have developed a chronic illness.

- We want to strengthen our self-esteem and a close friend makes a very offensive and disparaging comment.

- We want to find someone with whom we can have a serious, respectful and supportive relationship and all we get is indecent proposals from the supposedly high quality dating sites we registered for.

- We want to be listened to more and be treated with

more respect but our child, of all people, speaks rudely to us and dismisses everything we say.

- We want to begin to express ourselves more, feeling that we, too, have what to say and find ourselves silenced in several different situations.

## A reflection, training and internalization stop

In the aforementioned examples, we discuss both needs and desires, both conscious and subconscious, and every one of us has several dozen of these. This exercise is an invitation to stop for a moment, take a short pause and consider which events in our life, both large and small, both significant and ordinary, contained the element in which something entered our lives which looks exactly the opposite of what we wanted or that we thought we wanted. Recalling two or three such elements and practicing their identification and their deciphering at this time can help us significantly later on with internalization and imprinting of the insight on the practical level later on in our lives.

In the **first stage**, let us look at the event that we have just recalled and that is floating in the surface of our minds. Let us try, from a place of full honesty (spiced with a pinch of courage), to try to consider what might have been the true desire that led us to this event and what did we truly desire in our deepest heart of hearts?

In the **second stage**, in order to identify a costume (dear God, a roaring lion!) and pierce it to find the opportunity hiding beneath it (here is my chance to be brave), let us think the opposite of what arrived in practice, let us consider that: "We desired something and the opposite has happened." Then, let us see what floats to the surface, what is revealed. What was actually there behind the mask? Where did it come from and where has it taken us?

In the **third stage** we will imprint this insight, this magical "dropping of the other shoe," this blessed "Ahh!" moment by changing our perception of reality regarding this event from "This is the worst thing that had ever happened to us" to "This is one of the most significant things that has ever happened to us" to "Wow, this is a really incredible gift that we just received!"

*Want a few tricks?*

In order to dramatically shorten the time it takes us to recognize the opportunity, we can declare in advance that "This event is the perfect gift" and prepare a list of how this gift has contributed to our life.

If we do not truly believe this is a gift because there is part of us that is saying, "Oh, come on. A gift? Don't try to fool me." We can decide that we treat this task like a goal-oriented detective who must find a solution to the mystery because a human life depends on it. We are the detective and we must crack this mystery. We must locate this gift.

Another trick is to imagine that this event did not happen

to us but to a friend of ours. Imagine him in this event and to try to see what opportunity lies in wait for him in it. This detachment between us and the event / situation will help dissipate our emotional defensive screens, provide us with an additional perspective and increase clarity.

## The desires of the eternal spirit

Do you remember the spirit within us? This immortal and eternal part of which we may not be aware in everyday life but is nonetheless there, whispering, directing and speaking to us in super-creative ways (no less sophisticated than the costumes and disguises of the soul) while observing our lives from a bird's-eye view and relating to the lessons that we are here to learn? Remember how we said that awareness of the sophisticated "speech" of the spirit would lead us, as we progress in life from within this awareness, to identify the mechanisms that inhibit and promote our growth and to accept the changing circumstances of life as opportunities to develop?

Well, this is the opportunity to shed a light on the desires of this eternal and hidden aspect within us. **These desires, being separate of any physical body with desires and urges and also separate from an ego that is often unbalanced and does not fulfill its original intent (protection and survival), are linked to a supreme will.** This supreme will is linked to our destination, to the big picture, to the "What are we here for?" to the "What have we come here to experience?" to the "Why were we even born where we were born (geographically / politically), to the parents we were born to (how present and caring they were in our lives), the environment we grew up in (socio-economic condition, educational levels), family (supportive / approving / close / large), to culture (backward / progressive / goal-oriented / aggressive), to our body (internal and external characteristics) and circumstances (desired / planned pregnancy) in which we were born?" In our daily lives we rarely deal with these big questions because we are too busy dealing with the thousands of everyday daily tasks and with survival (existential- economic and psychological). The supreme will is not survival-oriented since it is not temporal and therefore, unlike our soul / ourselves, its existence is never threatened.

To summarize in two words the differences between the two types of desires the difference is in "vantage-point heights." *The desires of the eternal spirit are higher and deal with the big picture and the master plan, whereas those of the temporal soul are more grounded and deal with the minute details and the overload of daily life.* It can easily be seen that each part has its own desires and its own agenda. It may seem that they never meet and that they never can meet, that they are, in fact, polar opposites. How then can the complex mechanism called man operate, in spite of all of its contradictions?

Yes, the metaphysical spirit is incarnated in physical matter (a body that contains a soul). Yes, through matter, the spirit fulfills (or seeks to fulfill), itself. Yes, the spirit guides and directs the soul in many creative ways (just like the hidden passenger in the coach implants in the coach driver the coach's destination). Yes, the spirit evolves exactly as "we" do, through the physical-emotional experiences of the soul. Yes, the soul is a reflection of the spirit and it (and the body) were carefully selected in accordance with the supreme will and mission. And it appears that on the surface, the supreme choices (of the spirit) and the everyday choices (of the soul) are diametrically opposed. However, there is a meticulous plan in place that grants us the opportunity to choose differently, to change and to be changed -- even against all odds. There is here a complex and sublime combination of both supreme and earthly reasons. Even if we will not always know what the heights are (superior intellectual consciousness that create almost automatic understanding of "Why things are the way they are," for good or evil), the mere fact that they exist can ease how we face the hardships life.

*For the spirit, as with the soul, opportunities seem opposed to desires.*

Here are a few examples that illustrate how the supreme desires of the spirit are interwoven into the soul and the challenges.

- The spirit wants to explore and experience *self-control* so it chooses to materialize within a body-soul which deals with a type of eating disorder (lack of control over food) or a body-soul which deals with kleptomania (lack of control over the impulse to take something belonging to others) or a body-soul dealing with various forms of addiction (sex, drugs, smoking, alcohol, gambling...) or a body-soul which has been raised in a violent home and have themselves become a violent / abusive parent.

- The spirit wants to experience and explore *balance* which is why it will incarnate itself into a body-soul which is dealing with a bipolar disorder (rapid transition from depression to mania) or any other type of mental or physical disturbance that is expressed in imbalance or loss of balance.

- The spirit wants to experience and explore *faith*, which is why it will incarnate itself into a body-soul that is born into a religion hating atheistic home or else a body-soul which is physically paralyzed.

- The spirit wants to experience and explore *unity* which is why it will incarnate itself into a body-soul which is raised in a super xenophobic environment (be it racial, religious, nationalist or gender-based) or else in an environment which contains many contentious minorities.

- The spirit wants to experience and explore *self-acceptance* which is why it will incarnate itself into a body-soul that suffers from physical disability or physical limitations or else within a body-soul with unconventional or unusual appearance or even a transgender body (a dissonance between the gender identification of an individual and his biological gender).

- The spirit wants to experience and explore *self-worth* which is why it will incarnate itself into a body-soul that is growing up under abusive, humiliating or simply non-supportive parents who completely demolish its self-worth.

- The spirit wishes to experience *unconditional love* which is why it will incarnate itself within a body-soul that will give birth to a physically or mentally handicapped child (such as Downs syndrome, autism, muscular degeneration or mental retardation).

All of the aforementioned examples present starting positions in life that are seemingly the exact opposite of what the eternal spirit wishes to experience. This opposition is the opportunity to ascend beyond the autopilot, above the addiction, above the habits, above the disease, above all of life's varied circumstances and make a different choice.

This opposite is precisely what the spirit wants and this is how we have arrived at the *point of similarity and overlap between the polar desires of the temporal soul and the eternal spirit -- the mechanism of disguise. They both use it. Their desires might be polar opposites but their disguise mechanism is identical.* The mechanism of embodiment in matter / the reality of life and the manner in which they reach the opportunities to realize their desires is identical. Opportunities appear in disguise. So, even if we cannot know for certain whose desire (that of the spirit or that of the soul) is hidden behind this event which is occurring to us in reality, we can know for certain that there is an elaborate disguise at work here (which combines high level consciousness and the supreme reasons for action) and that there is an opportunity here for us. This knowledge, all on its own, can somewhat calm us, help us better accept the circumstances of life as a journey of development meant to bring us to a better place -- even if it currently looks and feels like the exact opposite.

**Alexander Graham Bell:**

*"When one door closes, another opens but we often look so long and so regretfully upon the closed door that we do not see the one which has opened for us."*

## *Summary of the first premise – opportunities appear in disguise*

- We are not always aware of what we truly desire of ourselves, of others or of life itself.

- Our true desire is hidden beneath opportunities that arrive at our door. If we learn how to identify this desire, we will learn how to exploit these opportunities to the fullest.

- The reasons to preferring the known difficulties over an unfamiliar opportunity include: Negative emotions, overwhelm reason and logic. We prefer to stick to the familiar, we are afraid of the unknown, our habits usually gain the upper hand and, critically, we fail to recognize the opportunities that arrive disguised in various costumes.

- The masks donned by the opportunities are cunning and can create considerable confusion since the opposite of what we seemingly want arrives. For example, we want to nurture and develop our courage and a terrifying lion arrives so that we will have the chance to overcome our fear and be brave.

- There is an "altitude gap" between the desires of the eternal spirit (which are independent of passions, urges, ego and supreme heights and dealing with the macro and the master plan) to the desires of the temporal soul (grounded and dealing with the micro and everyday life). This gap in altitude can cause considerable frustration.

- The mechanism of disguise is the overlapping point of similarity between the seemingly opposed desires of the temporal soul and the eternal spirit and both make use of it.

- There is a meticulous planning and a sublime integration of both earthly and supreme reasons (a higher consciousness which understands "Why things are as they are") which gives us the opportunity to choose differently, to change and be changed.

- Awareness of the sophisticated disguise mechanism of opportunities will help us accept the circumstances of our life as a journey of self-development that will bring us to a better place -- even if it looks and feels exactly the opposite.

# 2 Self-Compassion, Not Berating Oneself

*Welcome to jury duty*

Now that we've had a chance to get to know the sophisticated disguise mechanism of the opportunities which come knocking on our door, **we** will move on to the next premise which requires us to make a major modification to the autopilot application most of us adapt unthinkingly – self-berating ourselves. We will then try to move on to examine the circumstances of our life and the places where we are stuck from a viewpoint of self-compassion.

In the first chapter, when we considered the nature of the soul and compared it to the spirit, we saw that most of our thoughts are negative (a feature which is an evolutionary remnant from the prehistoric struggle for survival) and that we were no more than walking sacks of emotional waste that had accumulated throughout our life. This waste contains fear, anger, pain, guilt and shame. All of them together contain our reactions and how we think, speak and do things. In order to be able to still live and perhaps even enjoy life, we suppress, ignore, put on happy masks or swallow pills in order to suppress all of this unpleasantness (and even the depression) which occupies our bodies and our souls.

Since we are negative in our thoughts and emotions, we berate ourselves constantly. We berate ourselves, we judge ourselves and we criticize ourselves and do not give ourselves any credit or support. So does the environment (parents, relatives, colleagues, spouses, friends, partners). But, at some point in life we become the harshest critics of ourselves, as if something within us is telling all external judges and critics: "Guys, thank you for your years of selfless service, you really have done your work loyally over many years. Now, take some time off, have a cocktail on some exotic island and I will manage the judgment and criticism department. I promise you to toil day and night, without any sick days or time off and with very short lunch breaks."

Does this sound delusional? Does it sound like a joke? And yet, that is exactly how we behave without even being aware of it. Let's take a minute and consider  how many self-supportive thoughts do we have every day? How many pampering thoughts of encouragement and support that review our achievements (both external and internal) do we have every day? Without knowing any of you personally, I feel confident enough to guess that most of you probably cannot think of many or any. Now, take a moment to consider-how many self-critical thoughts we have every day? Thoughts such as: "What fuck ups / cowards / idiots / fools we are." "Nobody ever listens to us." "We don't have anything interesting to say about anything anyway." "How ugly / fat / stupid we are." "We never manage to do anything right." "No man / woman would ever want us." "We hate our body / face" and other such nuggets. How many times do these thoughts play repeatedly in our head, like a broken record, every day? Many, many times, right? It feels like the DJ overseeing these tunes can't be fired, right? So why is it like this? Why are most of us screwed up this way?

For the most part, we are this way because of the circumstances of our lives, lives in which we have been judged, insufficiently supported, criticized, humiliated, insulted, scared, hurt, shamed, angered, blamed and irritated by others from the moment we were born. At some point, we simply began to believe all of those unpleasant things different people throughout our life had repeatedly told us. Some of them thought they meant well by all of their criticism. They just wanted to protect us, to toughen us up and prepare us for real life. They really did care for us and most of them truly loved us, but each and everyone one of us had his personal pound of mud and slime smeared over him and this has consequences which are worth understanding. Before we rush to blame our parents and our environment for all of the trouble in our lives, even if it is true and they are responsible, it is important to clarify two things: Yes, our parents are the most important characters in the shaping of our conscious and unconscious mind. Yes, it is they who taught us about the world, how it works and how to operate within it. The worldview we inherited from them is the only one they knew -- they never knew anything else. Along the way, they may have also used or threatened physical violence against us. After all, over hundreds and thousands of years, and until quite recently, corporal punishment was an inseparable part of educating children. In order to achieve obedience – a beating or a ringing slap (or threats thereof) to maintain quiet -- a beating or a ringing slap (or threats thereof) to instill discipline -- a beating or a ringing slap (or threats thereof) to get respect -- a beating or a ringing slap (or threats thereof). That is how children were raised throughout most of history; that is how parents believed children should be raised and so that is why most parents did use corporal punishment. They did not know any other model of raising children. That is how they, themselves, were raised and that is how everyone around them was raising their children. If a parent had told a friend or a neighbor that his child was being unruly and that it was driving him nuts and that he did not know what to do with him, the most likely response would probably have been along the lines of: "If I were you, I would smack him once or twice. That will get him back on track." There would not have been, could not have been, any honest attempt to understand the source of that unruly behavior or its timing.

The second thing we must consider prior to blaming our parents for who we have become is related to a lack of awareness that was predominant until recent times, a lack of awareness regarding the destructive influence of words on children's emotions, behavior and character development. It is true that the proverb, "The tongue has the power of life and death" is ancient in origin (Proverbs 18: 21 -- based on King Solomon's musings) and it was well-known that words contain enormous power -- enough to create worlds from the void or destroy them. (That is why it is always recommended to "think before you speak" and oh, my, that is very hard advice to follow). Nonetheless, there was no true awareness of the terrible impact of unsupportive speech, humiliations heard and experienced, unsupportive words and repeated violence (be it physical, verbal or both) on a child's soul. Generally speaking, there was no awareness of the extent to which the words heard by our child on a daily basis, primarily but not exclusively at home, impact and shape the man he will grow up to be. Where do parents today get their greater awareness? In the past, people joked about how there were no parenting schools, that no one taught them how to be parents and that they simply learned from experience. But, in the present day, there are, in fact, parenting classes and even special parenting schools, and there is plenty of professional information available online. Today, there are groups and forums of parents, many schools and philosophies of parenting, TV programs concerning the issue and a wide variety of books. Our desire to be better parents than our parents were is now, thanks to all these, possible.

Today, we are aware of the fact that the majority of our beliefs, values, worldview and self-perception are etched into our subconscious (everything in our mind beyond the conscious) and by the age of seven. (The subconscious is like a sponge that soaks in all of our experiences in the world.) Later in our lives, we merely find "proof" that validates these beliefs, perceptions and conclusions about the world and ourselves. What are these beliefs, perceptions and conclusions? Exactly the neural wirings that form the pathway (and later the neural highways) we earlier discussed in our brain. These conclusions, beliefs and perceptions, utilizing these mental highways, become the glasses through which we experience and perceive reality. Sentences and phrases we have heard throughout our childhood such as: "What a screwed up child you are." "What did I do to deserve a trouble child like you?" "You will never amount to anything." "Maybe you better not even try, you will just be disappointed and your effort will be wasted." "You can try harder. Your best really isn't good enough." "I can't stand the sight / sound of you, get out of my face." "I don't understand how stupid a boy can be?" "Who would want to live with you to begin with?" "You are a constant source of embarrassment." "Everything you touch breaks." "You can't be trusted." "Haven't you understood yet that none of your infantile dreams will ever amount to anything?" "Why can't you be more like your brother / sister / neighbor's son?" "These sentences and others like them, or even one alone if it were repeated frequently enough, become our absolute truth. This "truth" accompanies us in every step we take, colors every thought we might have, turns us into who we are -- and we believe in it implicitly. We really are screwed up, we really are stupid, we really will not achieve anything in life, nobody wants to be with us and we truly are not worthy of anything. Each and every one of us can believe in any number as such "absolute truths" -- each deriving from one's own personal biography. That is how we constantly beat ourselves up -- because deep inside, we have over so many years believed these terrible things to be true. We believe that we truly deserve all of the evil / hardships / punishment / suffering we experience.

Of course, in addition to the impact of growing up as children in our parent's homes, there is also everything that happened to us afterwards -- as we grew up. All of the experiences, traumas and difficulties we were exposed to, both big and small, accumulated and were stored within us -- and all of them influence us today. It is reasonable to assume that a considerable portion of these experiences amount to validation or "proof" of the "absolute truth" that we are "screwed up" or that "something in us is just not right." Others will form the foundations of new beliefs, probably compatible to the "screw-up" that defines us. Maybe you think that you are all grown up and that none of the childhood nonsense of the past is relevant to us (after all, we survived, grew up and put it behind us) but, even if we have dug in behind reinforced concrete walls so that no one would ever harm us again (and that is why some of us feel nothing anymore -- neither the good nor the bad) be sure, be very sure, that even so the traumas of the past affect us, control us and manage us. Why? Because, as aforementioned, we are not much more than walking sacks of emotional waste accumulated over the years. That waste includes fears, anger, pain and guilt of all sorts -- which makes us bona fide experts in berating ourselves.

## Who wanted compassion and didn't get any?

All right, so berating oneself is the default autopilot for most of us. It is a six-lane (at least!) neural highway in our brain. Still, we saw in the previous chapter that if you so desire you can change anything, including the structure and the function of the brain. We saw that new pathways could be paved in the brain. So now is the time to ask: Why would we want to change our habit of beating ourselves up? What new habits do we want to exchange for it? My recommendation is that we exchange beating ourselves up with self-compassion. But hold on for a moment before you get your trusty machete out to blaze a new path through your mental jungle. First we need to define exactly what compassion is.

In the dictionary definition, "compassion" is a derivative of empathy which is typified by a desire to help another individual (to alleviate or lessen his suffering). This is the ability to feel the pain of the other out of a faith that he is capable of dealing with the situation, without your identifying with his pain, judging or pitying him. In simple terms, instead of judgment or criticism, we offer the other understanding and kindness when he fails or makes an error. So what is self-compassion? The same thing -- but towards ourselves -- when we are the ones who suffer, who fail or who feel unworthy, rather than berating ourselves with self-criticism (or suppressing / ignoring / fleeing the pain or the unpleasant feeling), to act with warmth and understanding towards ourselves.

Dr. Christine Nef,[6] one of the leading researchers in the study of self-compassion, recognized three components within it:

1. **Awareness** – A balanced approach towards our neg-

---

6      www.self-compassion.org (Neff, 2003) (Neff & Tirch, 2013.)

ative emotions so that we neither suppress them nor over-express them. (You cannot feel compassion towards pain while you ignore it.) It is saying, "It is hard for us right now / we are having a difficult time" instead of saying, "We are a failure / our life is insufferable / nothing happened / we don't want to think about it / we can't take it anymore."

2. **A common humanity** – Suffering and personal failure are part of the common human experience. Therefore, instead of thinking that everyone is doing well and only we are badly off, we must understand that it happens to everyone, not just us. It is like saying, "We are permitted to feel that way / it is natural to respond as we respond / we are not unusual" instead of saying that "We are nuts / screwed up / overreacting."

3. **Kindness to ourself**- Be kind and understanding towards ourselves when we suffer, fail or feel unworthy, instead of ignoring the pain or berating ourselves with self-criticism. It is saying, "We deserve a hug" instead of saying, "What idiots we are." It is important that we note that self-compassion is not self-pity such as "What poor sods we are" (being immersed in our own problems and forgetting that other people have similar problems). Nor is self-compassion self-alienation such as saying "Everything is fine," (although in practice we feel like shit). Nor is it giving ourselves a free ride, "Well, we are stressed so let's be nice to ourselves and

pamper ourselves with an entire box of ice cream." (After all, we want to be healthy and happy in the long run as well as in the short run.) Nonetheless, even if we find ourselves "all smelly in front of the television gorging ourselves on an entire family-sized pizza berating ourselves, this will certainly not get us anywhere or make us feel better about who we are in that moment in time. It is better to recognize that gorging ourselves in front of the TV is simply the best we can do at that moment but that we can and will, do better later on.

Now, let's put it all together and add the premise of "self-compassion instead of berating oneself" to the trilogy method and its three questions (which we will go over in part 3) and our desire to identify where we are stuck and what challenges we face, find out what lies beneath them and from there diagnose our situation and locate the path forward. If we choose to examine this challenging situation in our lives from a position of compassion towards ourselves, we will automatically be more honest, more open and even have slightly more courage to dive into our deeper layers and examine the situation as it truly is, without any disguise or stories (to justify the situation and therefore keep us safe) which our ego tells us to do. Perhaps, most importantly, thanks to this self-compassion, we will not feel under attack, helpless in the face of a stone-cold cruel firing squad. That in and of itself can assist us in achieving the higher perspective which we aspire to so that it might aid us when we come to analyze difficult situations.

Ronit Shefi Wolfin, a spiritual mentor, defines compassion as a state of mind which provides an answer to question: "Why are things the way they are?" Compassion is like a light lit in a dark room which shows the true shape of things. I will give a slightly radical example in order to illustrate this definition. If we run into a mother in the street or in a mall who is screaming at her child, and perhaps even threatening to slap him, our automatic response will be to judge and criticize her along the lines of "This is a terrible mother / the poor boy, this is heartbreaking / this is really bestial behavior to display in public / how can she humiliate her child like this?" and so forth. Some of us might even approach her and reprimand her for her inappropriate / disgusting behavior. However, what if someone had told us that this woman, only ten minutes ago, had discovered that her husband was cheating on her and having an affair with a younger woman? What if someone had come and told us that the woman's doctor had notified her, only ten minutes ago, that the tumor found in her breast was indeed malignant? What if someone had told us that this woman was unjustifiably fired from her job this morning and that her husband, unemployed for several months, had responded to the news with anger and shouting? Wouldn't we respond differently? Wouldn't we suddenly understand why she behaved as she behaved? Wouldn't we be more understanding? Wouldn't we immediately forgive her "disgraceful" behavior given the new facts which had come to light? Wouldn't we perhaps dare to ask ourselves how we would behave under similar circumstances? Wouldn't we put ourselves in her shoes and see that under such circumstances we would have acted in exactly the same way? Wouldn't we open up our hearts a little? This is the compassion that answers the question "Why are things the way they are?" This is the compassion which we must direct towards ourselves when we seek to diagnose ourselves (using the three trilogy questions) in hard, challenging, scary, unfair or embarrassing situations. When we are there, in the heart of the tornado, in that dark room, it is very scary because we cannot see anything (not even hope or the exit portal). This threatens and stresses us out. We are in a constant state of readiness and defensiveness (and therefore are prepared to be attacked at any given moment). We are curled into ourselves, are attentive to nothing but our fears, feel helpless, suffocated and perhaps our old victim mentality raises its ugly head again. ("Why do I deserve this?") And then, suddenly, someone presses the switch and turns on the light and we can see everything! Everything is illuminated; it all looks exactly the way it does without any masks or disguises. We can finally see the big picture in its entirety and details both large and small. And then, there is the Ahh! moment, the moment of pure understanding. It all finally comes together.

Self-compassion is the light; it is the torch which illuminates the dark room where we were and shows us things as they truly are. Self-compassion is what leads us and supports the "Ahh!" Now we finally understand why we act as we do / we finally understand why all this has happened / we finally understand why we failed." We yearn for this understanding because we know that it will lead us towards accepting the situation and will enable us to make the change and to break through the roadblocks and challenges which are impeding our progress. Research has indicated that self-compassion provides us with a feeling of emotional stability -- even in the face of failure -- and that, in and of itself, is a source of psychological resilience. In other words, self-compassion helps us to fear failure less; self-compassion enables us to deal with failure when it takes place and self-compassion makes us far more prepared to deal with the challenge, get up after falling down and proceed onwards.

## What about a personal example?

Below are a few personal examples from my own life with which I will illustrate how I taught myself self-compassion and how this helped me recover from various mental illnesses. Let me provide a short background. In my book, "Listen to your Soul and Heal your Body of Chronic Diseases" which includes an eight key guide for self-healing, I describe, among other things, my personal path of healing from seven diseases and illnesses, physical and mental, with which I was afflicted for many years (asthma, bulimia, bipolar disorder [manic-depression], hypothyroidism, migraines, ruptured disc and an addiction to light drugs) and how I reached my current healthy and balanced state in which no drug, medication or pills (or vomit inducing fingers for that matter) enter my throat. Teaching myself self-compassion occurred in the framework of two of the "healing and balance" struggles in which I was engaged -- weaning myself from light drugs and ending my binge eating and vomiting. My journey of healing lasted almost a decade. The first four years were dedicated solely to investigating the field of self-healing so that I might believe it was even possible to heal myself of physical illness (At that point I still concealed my mental illnesses from the world [and even myself] as I did not think it was possible to recover from them).

After seven years on my journey of self-healing (in which the latter three were the years in which I actively and vigorously pursued recovery from my physical illnesses -- asthma, hypothyroidism, migraines and disc ruptures), came a pivotal moment in which I was sitting in my yard, joint in hand and a powerful inner voice told me: "You know, you don't need drugs anymore. Now you are just addicted to them." At that moment, I knew deep inside that that voice was right and I understood what it was talking about. This point is important since at that time in my life, after 18 years of massive smoking of light drugs, I did not want to stop smoking them. I had fun with them. I liked them. They were an inseparable part of my life and my daily routine and just the thought of quitting made me shudder. Living my life without drugs wasn't even an option -- not in any parallel universe I could imagine. So why did I say that I knew that the voice was right and that I understood what it meant when it told me that "You don't need the drugs anymore?" Because the moment I heard those words the understanding that the drugs had fulfilled their purpose -- which was to protect me from my deep inner pain (and from anger, shame and guilt), the smokescreen through which I had lived my life and through which I saw the world was no longer necessary. The goal had been achieved and I could move on to the next stage of my life. But now, I had a physical addiction to deal with and to handle and it wouldn't be simple to get rid of it after so many years. But it was possible. For the first time in my life, joint in hand, I dared to think, "Well, it's time to stop doing drugs."

How long did it take from that pivotal moment to the day I was fully weaned off drugs and stopped puffing on an occasional joint? How long did it take to succeed? Three long years. Do you know how many falling off the wagon moments there are in three years? How many times I failed and found myself smoking again despite all the promises and despite my fierce desire to end my addiction? How many times was I disappointed with myself and berated myself for failing? Many, many times. "I'm fucked up." "Why am I doing this again?" "Why do I need this?" "I will never manage to stop harming myself again." "What do I have? How fucked up can I be?" "What a bummer I am." "I will never make it." "There is no way I can be without drugs." and other self-abasement phrases which led me to feel shitty about myself. One day I recalled the pivotal sentence I heard years before: "At any given moment an individual can only do the most he can do at that point in time." I began to implement it and remind myself of it every time I failed: "The best you can do right now is smoke the joint. Perhaps tomorrow you can make it, or the next week, or a month from now. Right now you can't." This was not giving myself a pass, this was self-forgiveness. I forgave my failure and I felt compassion for myself. Why wasn't this giving up? Because I did not choose to do nothing and merely hope that one day I would stop smoking drugs. In those years, I performed intensive healing work on four parallel channels (physical, mental, energetic and spiritual). I studied the sources of my addiction both on the level of my soul, with an emotional therapist, and on the level of my spirit, with a spiritual mentor. I mapped out the route that led to my addiction, learned to accept it, to understand it, to accept it and to forgive myself for it. That is why every time I failed, every time that I broke down and returned to puffing on my joints (and that would often occur after several months of staying on the wagon), I told myself that "This was the best I could do right now, to smoke the joint today and perhaps I will make it through the next day without one. Right now I can't." I supported myself. I paved a new pathway in my brain of self-compassion, a path which had never existed in the past, a path which with training and the years became a highway which replaced the happily neglected highway of berating myself. One day, at the right moment, it happened. I was completely weaned of my addiction.

## A finger down my throat...

This self-education took place in parallel to my vomiting. At that pivotal moment, holding my joint, I was in a place where I had already admitted to myself and to my emotional therapist who accompanied me, that I was a bulimic. I even made an effort during that period to quit the binge eating and vomiting rituals. On this front as well, every time I found myself over the toilet bowl pushing a finger down my throat and vomiting my guts out, I experienced considerable berating of myself and a great deal of self-hate. From the moment I recalled the supportive and compassionate sentence, I began to repeat it to myself every time I vomited: "The best you can do right now is push a finger down your throat. Perhaps tomorrow you can make it through without it or perhaps next week. Right now you can't." The more I repeated the sentence every time I fell off the wagon, the more I felt compassion for myself. Another factor which greatly helped me accept and understand my situation and hence feel greater self-compassion, were my studies with a spiritual teacher which, among other things, dealt with the earthly and supreme causes to this ongoing celebration of victimhood which contained both a pitiful victim and a vicious victimizer. Two for the price of one. We studied together why the spirit chose this life path and its eating disorder (a combination of "learning self-control" and "karmic residue") and where all of the self-hatred which led to this disorder came from. The combination of the spiritual studies, my fierce desire to get better and the application of self-compassion did its thing. One day, at the right moment, it happened. I was able to hold myself back in the middle of an eating binge because a very powerful and very insistent inner voice told me: "That's it. You are not shoving a finger down your throat ever again. Never. Stop your gluttony right now because your stomach is going to ache with so much food inside." And…I stopped. I swallowed the last bit in my mouth. Since it was evening, I went to bed with a very unpleasant feeling, with two holiday meals stuffed into my single stomach but with the certain knowledge that there would be no more vomiting and that I would never harm myself like that again. So it is true that I never shoved a finger down my throat again and I never dared shove such insane quantities of food into my body either. But it still took me two years to successfully balance my residual emotional feeding -- eating junk food, candy and all sorts of sweets. (Every evening I had to consume several spoons of Nutella chocolate spread.) I was eating out of boredom and I was eating due to my emotions (fear, anger, sadness, shame, guilt….). The spoonfuls of Nutella chocolate spread was no conscious choice to "pamper myself a little" but an uncontrollable urge. I would tell myself: "This is the best you can do right now. You cannot control it, not just yet. Perhaps tomorrow you will be able to or perhaps next week." One day I noticed that for several evenings I had not gone to the cabinet where the Nutella jar was. I had ended my uncontrolled and harmful behavior. I had managed to restore my self-control in the field of food and the self-compassion which replaced the berating of myself had a very significant role in this process.

---

## A reflection, training and internalization stop

If the stories above have touched you and you wish to start to develop general compassion or self-compassion or to amplify them, here are three tips that can help you in this task:

**Developing general compassion**
*Imagining harsh circumstances* – If there are any individuals in your environment whom you tend to judge, whose actions

or behavior you tend to criticize or just constantly irritate you, if you want to do something and change the situation, imagine that you have just found out that this individual has just received terrible news (a terrible illness / spousal betrayal / the death of a loved one) and that this is the reason he behaves as he does. Perhaps you cannot change the irritating individual, but you can change your reaction towards him ("given the difficult circumstances" your reaction will be more compassionate, caring and calm). That, in and of itself, will lead you to feel better about yourselves. For the truly dedicated, trying to imagine these harsh circumstances might motivate you to do something you had never imagined you would do, offer help to this individual, show an interest in his condition and ask if there is anything you can do to help him. Go figure out where this road might lead you. You will certainly feel better once you are there.

**Nurturing self-compassion**

*Practice the compassionate sentence* – Every time you find yourself performing the action you wish to quit (smoking, drinking, gorging, self-harm or any other uncontrolled behavior), tell yourself: "This is the best I can do at this time point. Perhaps tomorrow I can do better, perhaps the day after that, perhaps next week and perhaps only in a year. At the moment, this is simply the best I can do." Try to add an additional channel of treatment / activity which will support taking back control such as emotional therapy, a support group, expanding your knowledge on the subject of your difficulty or sharing your problem with someone close by asking for his help and support.

**Separate yourself from the situation** -- Imagine that anything that is happening to you (smoking, drinking, overeating, self-harm or any other uncontrollable behavior) is happening to someone else, is happening to your best friend who you truly love. Then imagine that this friend is sharing his self-harming actions with you and how hard it is to him and how he berates himself for being so weak. What would you tell him to support him? What would you tell him to cheer him up? What would you tell him to make him feel better about himself? Now dare to say these very same things to yourself. You are no less worthy of this support and understanding.

## Summary of the second premise -- self-compassion instead of berating oneself

- This premise is a chance to move on to examine the circumstances of our life and the places where we are stuck from a position of self-compassion rather than one of self-understanding.

- At some point in our lives, we have become the harshest judge of ourselves and we are berating, criticizing, belittling and not supporting ourselves.

- Throughout our lives we have been criticized, we have been humiliated, we have been shamed and accused and, at some point, we simply began to believe all of these terrible things about ourselves. We came to believe that we deserve all the evil / difficulties /

punishments / suffering we encounter.

- Until recent times, people were unaware of the destructive consequences of words on emotions, behavior and the character of an individual.

- Conclusions, beliefs and perceptions, through the neural pathways in our brain where they are repeatedly applied, become our "absolute truth" which operates us and becomes the lenses through which we perceive and comprehend reality. We believe it.

- Self-compassion – when we suffer, fail or feel unworthy, we treat ourselves with understanding and kindness rather than berating ourselves with self-criticism (or else suppressing, ignoring or fleeing the pain and the unpleasant feeling).

- Compassion is the way to answer the question "Why are things the way they are?" and it is like the torch shining a light into a dark room and showing us the true shape of things.

- Examining challenging situations in our life from a place of self-compassion also enables greater honesty and openness (which grants us the courage to dive into deeper layers) as well as the development of a spiritual perspective.

- Self-compassion gives birth to understandings which lead us towards accepting the situation. And that, in and of itself, enables us to make the change and to exit the blocked up or challenging condition.

# 3 Every Setback Is an Opportunity for Growth

*Everything in the universe grows, not just plants*

What all living things in the universe, large and small, have in common is a desire to grow and to evolve, to expand and to develop, regardless of whether they are plants, animals or the universe itself as a whole. We grow, and as we grow we change to accommodate this growth. Whatever does not grow, whatever stays in one place, withers, dies, or smells and rots (exactly like still water that does not flow). We humans, the crown of creation (no matter that there are those who argue, justifiably, that we are pretty rotten at that job) are no exception when it comes to growth. It is only when growth takes places, not only physically, as it is with the plant world or physically and emotionally, as it is in the animal world, (yes, of course animals feel emotions) but on four different levels. We will begin with the first which is the most apparent to the eye -- *physical growth*. This growth begins the moment that we are created by the interaction of an ovum and sperm. The union between them creates a cell that constantly divides and continuously grows until the final product that is called a baby – pure and a screamer -- is created. This cute baby, from the moment he is born, physically grows and develops into a child, a teen, a man, a woman. At some point the withering process begins. The stage of old age arrives and then the completion of his role in this life and the retirement from the physical world. This same process of growth withering, aging, death also characterizes the plant kingdom and the far richer and more diverse animal kingdom.

Moving on to our *psychological growth*. This is composed of two channels -- emotional and mental growth. They, too, it seems, begin even as we swim in our mother's womb. There are countless studies from all over the world which have studied the issue and show that as embryos we have capabilities (such as memory, capacity to learn and the ability to adapt to our environment),[7] that they have needs, that they think, feel and are responsive to the environment.[8] Moreover, events which we experience in the womb are etched into our memory

---

7        Memory has been studied via three learning processes: Conditioning, adaptation and exposure. All of the researchers reached the same conclusion: An embryo has memory and has a capacity to learn (Leader 1991, Hepper 1992). A study that discusses the embryonic source of illness in adults has found that embryos that suffered from delays in in-utero growth had a higher chance of falling ill after their birth with such diseases as excessive blood pressure, coronary artery obstruction, obesity and diabetes (Barker, 1993).

8        A researcher by the name of Giannakoulopoulos proved, in 1994, a laboratory finding that confirmed pain in endorphin levels in an embryo's blood. Embryos also display goal-oriented movement -- for example, if during amniotic fluid sampling the

(subconscious memory) and can even affect our lives after we are born.[9]

As we have seen, *mental growth* precedes our birth into this world. From the moment we are conceived, through our birth

---

needle touched them, they withdraw, and if bitter substances were injected into the amniotic fluid, they ceased swallowing.

In short, there is early intelligence that enables the embryos to distinguish between stimuli that benefit them and stimuli that do not (like little children or animals which "know" which stranger they should approach and which they should avoid). Embryos have the ability to identify hands placed on their mother's stomachs! Certain embryos approach and move at the touch of one individual and "freeze" at the touch of another individual.

It has been proven that as of week 23, REM sleep (rapid eye movements indicating dreaming) occurs in embryos. This is a type of sleep which requires mental and even emotional activity.

Dr. *Alessandra Piontelli* has studied the issue of embryo temperament and found that continuity exists between embryonic life and the post-natal period and that embryos have very similar temperaments to what they display after birth. The results of the study are detailed in her book "From Fetus to Child" (1992).

9        Three psychological therapists, Frank Lake, Stanislav Grope and Athniseus Kafkalides, from Britain, the Czech Republic and Greece respectively, who were not familiar with each other, used LSD when treating their patients (back then it was permitted and even common) and thereby enabled their patients to recall memories from being embryos and from their birth. In many cases these experiences were then verified with the patients' mothers, indicating that the memories were true and not drug induced hallucinations.

and to the moment we die, we are constantly learning. At first, we learn how to behave, beginning at the most basic level such as eating, diaper changes, receiving a smile from its mother and understanding what needs to be done in order to spend as much time as possible in mommy's arms. We learn how to crawl, how to walk, the social space surrounding us (who is responsible for which activities and which actions lead to the desired or undesired results). We learn how to manage ourselves in this space and how to get what we want. Slowly the social circle broadens from mommy-daddy, to the wider family, to the environment and to the world. We are curious and want to know more and more, not necessarily in the framework of school, but at any time and in any place. We are passionate about this learning and are filled with enthusiasm when we learn something new. We study a profession or gain a higher education, work, create, act to achieve our next target or goal and move on. At some point in life we grow a bit tired (children, mortgage, endless stress and non-stop bombardment 24/7 of information, most of it negative and depressing) of learning new things. Nonetheless, whether we want to or not, we keep on learning and accumulating new information. Life and circumstances do not give us any other option. The very fact that we open our eyes up to a new day leads us to think, act and develop mentally (each one of us, of course, at his own pace and with his own unique characteristics.

**Emotional growth** also starts in the womb. We experience a wide range of emotions, in accordance to what our mother experienced (sorrow, anger, fear, stress, joy and enthusiasm), in accordance with the environment in which she is (supportive or otherwise) and depending on whether our pregnancy was planned or, more accurately, on whether we were desired or not. (An extreme example from the field of criminology:The study involved a population of particularly violent individuals. It was found that their mothers had attempted to abort them but that the abortions failed for some reason and they survived. Crazy, right?)

At first, the horizons of our emotional world are very narrow. All we care about is ourselves; all we want to do is feel as "good" as possible and so every little thing disturbs our calm (just try taking candy from a child. Welcome to the nightmare vision of the apocalypse -- that is exactly what he is emotionally experiencing). As we age and develop, we become more and more aware of our environment and the fact that others also have feelings. We learn how to share (and give up the "This is mine, I don't want him to have it.") and learn how to be more aware of our own emotions --though not nearly as much as we should. This is partly because we are taught that it is impolite to freely express our negative emotions and partly because it is simply easier to suppress or stew in our negative emotions. Acknowledging them is often too painful and unpleasant. As the years go by, most of us open our hearts more and more (each in accordance to his own capabilities) and the parents among us know exactly what it is all about because our children, seemingly cruelly (through sleepless nights and hours long weeping), force us to be more patient, more accepting, more giving and far more attentive than we were before parenthood. We feel much more and are significantly less egotistical, self-centered than we were before parenthood.

Once we reach our post-retirement golden years, we are generally far calmer, less excitable, more compassionate, more forgiving and more loving. A lovely example of this is grandparents who sense a type of "parenthood second opportunity" feeling wildly insane love for their grandchildren that they lacked, at least in these dosages and power, when they were young and raised their own children. That is why many of them proclaim that loving one's grandchildren is an unparalleled experience, something completely different from anything else. This is due to a nice combination of environmental conditions which make this love possible (less pressure, less responsibility, less accumulated fatigue and much more free time) with the heart being opened up sufficiently to enable people who were shut up / closed off / uptight / stiff / tightly wound all of their lives to prance about like children in the grass or in the playground and to permit their grandchildren to ride them, pull their hair and kick their heels into their ribs. This opening of the heart also allows them to accept the other, the different and perhaps even the despised from the past (a classic example is the acceptance of grandchildren and / or spouses from undesired, unaccepted and even shunned marriages).

## *Can one grow metaphysically as well?*

*Energetic growth is also related to raising our frequency, the frequency at which all of our cells and the molecules and the atoms in our body vibrate.* This frequency can be measured with scientific tools, so this is not "spiritual stuff" but basic facts of physics. We are not nearly as solid as we perceive ourselves to be. It may sound nuts but when we get down to the level of the particles which make up seemingly solid matter to molecules and then to atoms, we discover that atoms are no more than a hollow sphere of energy at the center of which is a tiny nucleus made up of even tinier particles (they are like whirlpools of energy rotating around each other) and around the nucleus electrons rotate at an enormous distance (relative to the size of nucleus). The atoms are actually 99.99999% space and they vibrate. Every such hollow and vibrating sphere of energy is connected to another such hollow and vibrating sphere and so on. That is how the molecules, which also vibrate and make up solid matter, are formed. That is what we are made up of. Simply put, the seemingly solid matter in our universe is not solid at all, it is made up of energy and that energy vibrates at a certain frequency. We ourselves are vibrating creatures and every one of us vibrates at a certain frequency. You can measure the frequency of anything in nature (frequencies are measured in Hertz units with which we are familiar from the world of sound). Our thoughts and emotions also have frequencies. Negative thoughts or sensations such as shame, anxiety, sadness, anger and hatred have frequencies around 0-200 Hertz. In contrast, positive emotions or sensations such as optimism or joy have higher frequencies in the 600-Hertz range (the frequency measured and attributed to Love is 528 Hertz and it is a much-studied frequency.[10]

In other words, *a good feeling has a high frequency and a bad feeling has a low frequency*. We are affected by the frequencies of others in the environment around us and this is easily apparent. When an individual is angry and nervous, this automatically influences everyone in his environment. If a parent is raging all over the home, the atmosphere in the entire home feels so tense that a knife can slice it. The opposite is true as well. Spend time with a happy, optimistic and easy going individual or even a smiling baby and their frequency will affect ours and our mood will rise. His frequency will pull our own frequency up. *Frequency / energetic growth leads us to adapt a high, stable and continuous frequency, not just in specific circumstances but all the time*. We do our best to bring ourselves to a point where we feel good about

---

10      The 528 Hertz frequency, also known as the "love frequency" or the "transformation frequency," exists at the mathematical level in every frequency of every living and growing thing on this planet. Furthermore, it is known as a frequency that returns human DNA to its original pristine form and geneticists and biochemists have been using it for years to repair and heal DNA in labs all over the world. It is one of the frequencies belonging to the musical solfeggio musical scale which includes nine frequencies considered part of the sacred geometry from which the universe is constructed. The solfeggio musical scale is a term struck by Dr. Leonard Horowitz and Dr. Joseph Puleo in their 1999 book, "Healing Codes for the Biological Apocalypse."

ourselves over time. And yes, this is work that requires dedication and perseverance leading to the formation of new neural pathways. But it is worth it. Regularly inserting things which make us feel good about ourselves (a walk in nature, dancing, purifying heart-to-heart conversations, creativity, a hobby, self-expression and more), together with work on our awareness (investigating ourselves and developing self-awareness) and emotional work (cleaning up our emotional waste) will lead us to development and change and growth to the next level. In other words, mental and emotional growth lead to energetic growth.

Our spiritual growth actually combines the three types of growth detailed here, together with awareness and connection to the spirit, connection to that eternal (and primarily hidden) part within us which speaks (or more accurately whispers) and communicates with us in a very sophisticated manner (through feelings and intuitions, conditions in reality, dreams, pains and illnesses, gut feelings and intuitions, ideas which "suddenly" appear in our minds and powerful epiphanies of the heart). In the first chapter we saw that a man who grows spiritually also develops, by necessity, emotionally, and in his awareness and hence energetically as well (because his frequency generally rises). We have also seen that if he implements his spiritual knowledge in the circumstances of his life, recognizes the various layers of his soul and identifies the growth promoting and growth inhibiting components in him, this will gradually lead him to accept the circumstances of his life out of the understanding that they contain a lesson that is meant to take us to the next step in our development. This, in and of itself, generates more serenity, more desire to create and fulfill ourselves, greater activism (initiative) and less reactivity, more self-attentiveness and awareness of our true desires, more control over our thoughts and their silencing and yes, also greater health and calmness.

## *What about when we cease growing and get stuck?*

All of the above regarding growth is good and well and it seemingly appears that all this is a euphoric sequence of events occurring in some ideal utopian world where we just grow and grow. Everything is sparkling and calm and everything is serene. All is illuminated and the path ahead is well-paved. But that is not how things work in the real world, is it? In reality, we are not plants whose highlight of the day is photosynthesizing the light of the sun or animals living in the wild and having no care other than locating prey to devour and mates to breed with, right? We are human beings with mortgages and children. We are stressed, we have it rough, we are in pain, we experience various losses and we are angry, depressed or occasionally despairing. We are scared and terrified of the next terror attack, the growing debit in the bank or the virus that the kid in kindergarten just caught. We are ashamed of many things we are, that we have done or that were done to us. We feel guilty or victims or both and, in general, we are rather negative most of the time, even if this negativity is not our fault. That is why we suffer considerably and we are rather stuck in that pain and fail to evolve (there is a very high correlation between negative feelings and emotions to be being stuck. When we do not feel well, we feel heavy and lack any motivation to go anywhere or to do or to change anything. When we are feeling optimistic, we are lighter (higher frequency), open to ideas and the world, optimistic and therefore more spontaneous-creative-active-fulfilling-developing).

*So what happens when we are stuck*? What happens when, for a very long time, we tread water and fail to develop? Well, have no fear. Life and the universe will give us a slight push. In fact, they will do everything to get us out of our comfort zone (including, in extreme situations, when that comfort zone is that pool of shit that we have simply gotten used to and even fond of). Life will encourage us to keep on developing. So the opportunities to do so will turn up. Guess what? We will not even recognize some of them because they will appear disguised as something else.

We need to realize that the supreme desire of our spirit is no different than the principle of growth common to all living beings. Its sole desire is to learn, grow and develop, even though it seemingly has "all the time in the world" being an eternal entity which does not suffer from stress or is forced to work with an hourglass. Therefore, it will create for us the conditions, situations and events that will force us to halt the race of life, reflect, choose another path, force us to change and force us to learn, grow and evolve. When we do, and when our spirit is satisfied, we will feel it on the physical level, the mental-cognitive level and the emotional-soul level. We will know it in every bone of our body simply because we will feel better about the situation and ourselves and from this place we will begin to internalize that *every setback is a chance for growth*. There are not any good or bad things happening to us, just different types of opportunities for growth, learning and development.

Yes, that is certainly hard to accept when we are in pain. It is hard to hear when we are suffering; it is hard to hear when we aren't feeling well. It is hard to hear when we fail; it is hard to hear when we are slapped on the face by reality. It is hard to hear when we are scared; it is hard to hear when we are insulted and it is hard to hear when it seems the whole world is against us. It is no less hard to hear when all of the aforementioned is happening to our friends and loved ones. However, that does not make it any less true or relevant to us. That is simply the way things work down on this planet. You grow, evolve and learn, primarily by facing challenges and hardship. The sooner we learn how to accept and internalize this, the less we will suffer and the more we will be able to honestly analyze the situation from a higher spiritual perspective and thereby arrive at solutions that are more precise and more connected to our true essence. Only then will we be able to help ourselves get unstuck with greater rapidity and with less suffering.

## Two supporting axioms

So how do you do it? How do you begin to accept and internalize the premise that "Every setback is an opportunity for growth" even when we are feeling bad and shitty? How can we create this new neural pathway in our brain? The solution proposed here is to recite day and night the following two supporting axioms: "*Whatever comes my way comes to develop me*"[11] *and "Whatever rises to the surface, rises on its way out." The first axiom relates to various situations that reality throws at us and the second refers specifically to negative emotions.* Together, these axioms provide us with direction, precision and understanding of what is happening to us and what we feel in regards to what is happening to us. They also help us to *reduce and dull the emotional pain* without resorting to chemicals (or other external substances such as painkillers, alcohol or drugs) or transferring the emotional pain to physical pain in the form of self-hurt (such as etching the skin with a knife).

"*Whatever comes my way, comes to develop me.*" At the base of this axiom which refers to situations reality throws at us, we understand that suffering, failure and the absence of perfection are part of the overall human condition. In other words -- it happens to everyone and we are not the only "fuckups"-- even if it feels like it sometimes. That, in and of itself, is somewhat helpful and empowering, helping us to accept our situation-- our experience is shared by others. Although each has his own particular experiences, we all go through the same basic experience. *In the next stage, we must connect the failures we experience into the process of our development.* Yes, we hate to

---

11    From the "The simplicity in Divinity" by the Louharya center

fail; we are afraid to fail. We can listen to the success stories of thousands of different people who will share the many, many failures they suffered on the road to success, including Thomas Edison who had to burn 10,000 light bulbs until he was able to develop the first successful electric light bulb ("I didn't fail. I merely found ten thousand ways that do not work") or the successful and sought-after actress who attended hundreds of auditions over the years where she was repeatedly told that with her looks she had no chance in Hollywood. All we will recall is their final crowning success -- the light bulb which shone or the Oscar award. *Some of us may already know in our head that failure is part of the path to success but we aren't really prepared to feel this failure in our heart because it makes us feel like a failure.* (Indeed, even the small, everyday failures we experience remind us of this painful fact and show us how unwanted or unworthy we are.) It is not a good place to be, not at all. We do not want to be there. The key is to approach this point from our hearts, think it from the heart and understand it from the heart. Everything that is happening to us is meant to develop us, or else it would not have happened to us. That is how we can transform around the equation:

**"Failure = shame = pain"**

**to**

**"Failure = learning = development = growth"**

If we do turn this equation around, our pain will diminish. As it diminishes, we will be able to learn more from these situations and from these failures and feel better about ourselves as we do and walk away from each failure with our heads held up high.

## "*Whatever rises to the surface, rises on its way out*"

The basis of this axiom[12] relating to our emotions is the understanding that the entire spectrum of emotions is legitimate since they all teach us something about ourselves. Not only the positive, fun and hip emotions we really enjoy but also the negative, painful and difficult emotions from which we run away or that we suppress. Our positive emotions teach us that we are exactly at the right place for this specific time. They teach us that the present moment is precisely right for us. It may be that the situation will change in another minute or another fifteen minutes but, in this specific time, it is precisely right for us and we do not need to do anything else. The negative emotions are a completely different story for one very simple reason – there is a hidden and yet untold story in them. Whether we want to hear it or are ready to hear it is a completely different story. In other words, *negative emotions and pain are like giant torches directed inwards, inviting us to enter deep within ourselves*. They themselves can also hint as to the origin of this emotion and where we can locate it -- if we begin to pay attention to its timing. When do we feel this emotion? In what place do we feel it? Is this situation something that repeats itself in our lives? Who is making us feel this

---

12      Taken from the lectures of the spiritual mentor Michael Assedo.

way? In what places or situations do we feel this emotion? The answers to these questions are the first key you need to answer the question "Why do we feel so badly at the moment?"

This is the place to note yet again that each and every one of us (without exception) is a walking sack of accumulated emotional waste. This waste is composed of countless places in our soul that experienced pain and suffering and have not yet received a proper remedy. These emotions rise and float to the surface, appearing as our negative automatic feelings so that they might receive this remedy, in order to cleanse them and free them so that we may be freed from them. Therefore, while it is true that our autopilot tries to evade pain because it hurts, we must understand that if we agree to pass through these painful places, the passage will purify us and help us grow and develop. These emotions would not rise if we lacked the maturity to handle the issue with a more mature, experienced, and wiser outlook – in better circumstances than in which it occurred in the past.

For example, if we feel rage at a given situation, this rage is already part of us. It has been part of us for a long, long time. This rage is an old one, not a new one. It is merely that the circumstances we currently experience have led it to arise. Therefore, the basic concept is to use exactly this situation to tell ourselves, "*Whatever rises to the surface, rises on its way out.*" In other words, we understand that this rage has existed within us for a long time and it now wishes to purge itself from us. In the *first stage,* it will be easier for us to accept it and ourselves in this situation. Perhaps we can even feel greater compassion towards ourselves for feeling or acting in rage instead of being angry or disappointed with ourselves. We will understand that this rage has a "valid inner cause," not just seemingly minor external circumstances that triggered it. **In the second stage**, we will be required to ask the following questions: What is really making me angry? Who is making me angry? When else am I so angry? When in my past have I been so angry? The answers will provide us with direction to the place within us that is in pain and is seeking solace. Merely reaching that spot, recalling it and the emotion that was involved in it, can provide us with the required answers. **In the third stage,** in order to release and purge the pain and / or rage underlying our response to the situation, we will simply feel it again. But this time, we will go through it from a wiser, more self-aware place, until it fades away and is expelled from us. This is because this pain has a purpose, it has a specific goal -- it is a pain of liberation and of healing. The very same place within us that has been broadcasting distress signals through this rage has received the attention and the response it required and we, being wiser, more experienced, more mature and more accepting than in the past, can supply this response. Cleaning these particles of emotional debris, one particle at a time, transforms us over time into lighter individuals (a heavy emotional burden has been lifted) and our perception of the world is slowly transformed into a brighter and more positive one, just as if we had removed negative glasses with which we have been experiencing the world from our eyes.

So, tying it all together, it is highly recommended you practice the two axioms "Whatever comes my way, comes to develop me" and "Whatever rises to the surface, rises on its way out" for every encounter or incident or information or emotion which enters or shows up in our life, dozens of times each day. Seriously. Call it "positive brainwashing" meant to help us separate and disconnect ourselves from the automatic suffering and negativity. As aforementioned, this world was designed to help us evolve, learn and grow -- primarily through the experiences (mental and emotional) , which are hidden in the challenges and hardships. We can address complaints to the big boss who designed and created this operating system or else we can just learn to accept and work with this operating system, gradually reduce the intensity of the pain, examine these situations with wisdom, sensitivity and honesty and from there, reach more precise solutions which will help us get unstuck or get over the challenge / obstacle / difficulty more rapidly and with less suffering along the way. Give it a try and allow the results to speak for themselves.

*Summary of the third premise – Every setback is an opportunity for growth*

- All things in the universe, large and small, grow and evolve -- plants, animals, humans or the universe itself.

- In human beings, growth occurs in four parallel layers: *Physical growth* (growth-growing old-dying), *psychological growth* which is composed of two channels of growth: *Mental growth* (learning to accumulate knowledge from the circumstances, experiences and events of our lives) and *emotional growth* (learning how to relax, forgive and primarily open up our hearts to ourselves and the environment), *energetic growth* (learning how to raise and stabilize our frequency as much as possible since such a high frequency is accompanied by a positive feeling) and *spiritual growth* (combing the three other types of growth with the connection to the spirit -- our eternal and hidden part).

- *When we are* stuck, stand in place and do not develop, we get a little push from reality. Life will try to get us out of our comfort zone and will create for us situations, events and conditions that will force us to stop, reflect and change. We will be forced to grow.

- It is recommended you recite two supporting axioms daily: *"Whatever comes my way, comes to develop me"* (refers to situations reality throws at us) and "Whatever rises to the surface, rises on its way out" (refers to negative emotions). Together, they provide us with a cerebral and emotional understanding of what is happening to us and they help us reduce the emotional pain we feel.

- If we can take to heart the axiom that everything that happens to us is designed to help us evolve, we can transform the equation "failure = shame = pain" to the equation "failure = learning = growth" and thereby reduce our pain and increase our wisdom.

- *Negative emotions and pain are like giant torches aimed inwards,* inviting us to discover the painful story behind them. *In the first stage,* it will be easier for us to accept ourselves in this situation. *In the second stage,* we will ask questions so as to get direction to the place within us that is in pain and seeking a response. *In the third stage,* in order to release and purge that pain, we will feel it repeatedly and pass through it until it fades. This is a pain with a defined purpose and goal, a pain of release and healing.

- Cleaning up the particles of emotional waste within us, one particle at a time, transforms our worldview into a more positive one, as if we removed negative lenses from our eyes.

# The Three Trilogy Questions

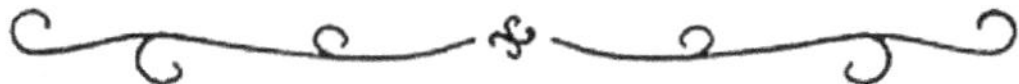

## Where is the silver lining in the cloud?

## Why did we create this situation?

## What can we change?

**The three trilogy questions:**

1. Where is the silver lining in the cloud?
2. Why did we create this situation?
3. What can we change? (in thought, emotion and deed)?

After we investigated and examined the special relationship between the three parts of man (temporal body and soul and eternal spirit), we defined the premises that form a mental-conceptual foundation of the trilogy system. It is now time to familiarize ourselves with the three questions that form the operational heart of the trilogy system. The first two questions are a sort of theoretical-conceptual preparation for the third, practical question. The first question is "Where is the silver lining in the cloud?" It is the easiest to answer of the three. The second question, "Why did we create this situation?" is the hardest and requires a great deal of self-compassion in order to receive a precise and honest answer. Answering both questions at once leads to the practical solutions which the third question, "What can we change? (in thought, emotion and action)" provides.

This is a chance to uncritically and non-judgmentally examine what rises to the surface while, at the same time, carefully examine the automatic resistance that arises within us at the questions (and be certain that they will arise, particularly at the second question). Why should we carefully examine them? Since this resistance poses in and of itself and hints to the solution to the third question -- like giant flashlights directed at the treasure we seek. This is the place to remind ourselves to wear self-compassion glasses while we process the resulting information. Our goal is not to suffer beyond what we are already suffering or to pour oil on the bonfire of negative emotions. Nor is it the goal to identify the guilty party responsible for our situation and point an accusing finger at it (nor to our reflection in the mirror). That is because the goal is not to, once again, berate ourselves. Our only purpose is to shine a light on this oppressive emotional darkness, see where we are stuck, receive valuable insights and thereby ease three important fronts: The mental front, the emotional front and the behavioral front. We must be brave, honest and open. Most importantly, we must open up our hearts.

# 1 Where Is the Silver Lining in the Cloud?

This important question is positive and joyful in its essence -- even when it deals with situations and events that are defined by us as difficult, harsh and even cruel. This important question, though it may be regarded or seen as simple, contains many different layers that we will examine. However, the most important thing to understand in regard to this question is to understand that *any "bad" event or situation you might encounter hides something good within it. Every cloud has a silver lining,* as corny as it may sound. Yes, sometimes that silver lining is not on the surface of the event or situation and you need to look deeply in order to see or find it -- but be certain that it is there.

The question "Where is the silver lining in the cloud?" *actually forces us to be positive, forces us to leave the negativity that we are accustomed to* -- even if we are not aware of this negativity or fail to notice it and believe that we are essentially optimistic people. *This question forces us, like a pistol to our temple, to find the potential for growth* that we discussed in the previous chapter, in the discussion of the third premise. Why is such "violence" required, you might ask? For a very simple reason: Because otherwise we would fail to do this. We would not lift our heads to look beyond and above this hard or painful situation precisely because we are in pain and because things are difficult. When we are in pain, we are "on the dark side of the moon" and we do not feel like leaving it or even trying too hard to see the light on the other side. Some of us will even be angry at the very idea. This includes such difficult situations in life such as a difficult disease, an accident, a traumatic event such as a divorce, a rocking betrayal, being fired or a life-shaking death of someone dear to you. However, it also includes supposedly easier situations that contain suffering which are easier to bear. That suffering is still there, part of the package deal that is life and includes various aches and pains, failures in everyday tasks, hurt feelings, being lectured or scolded, lies, verbal or physical violence, rage outbreaks and so forth. We feel pain in both the harshest and the easier situations and therefore our automatic response in such moments is to focus on the pain and to feel self-pity. We do not really control this response and it is exactly for this reason that this essentially "positive and exultant" question pops up which is seemingly not related to anything, seeking after the unseen benefit in this situation -- even if it is hidden from view. It is there, just waiting to be found.

## Our supreme good, not our immediate good

Another layer of this question deals with our supreme good, a basic principle of action here on this planet. It is part of our operational software. Our supreme good is the "big picture" good. It is concerned with the long run rather than the short, with our growth and development (mental, psychological, energetic and spiritual). It interweaves the individual with the collective good. That is to say, it extends beyond the boundary of the "me" and crosses into the territory of "we" (on the level of a couple, a nuclear or extended family, a department in work, the level of your building / street / neighborhood / city / state, the level of your profession and so forth).

This principle is incredibly frustrating and even annoying, particularly when you are in pain and when the going gets rough. This is because our supreme good is usually the opposite of our immediate good. Right now, all we want is some peace and quiet because the din is so loud we can barely hear ourselves. What we want right now is that the pain (be it psychological or physical) stop, never mind developing and evolving beyond them. What we want right now is to know "what will be?" because we are confused and the absence of clarity is driving us nuts. Right now we want a promotion and the idiot that we hate just got it. Right now we want to go on a vacation and this is not possible. Right now we want a date with the object of our affections but he does not want us like we want him. Right now we want to break into a certain field and we just cannot seem to succeed. That "right now" is our immediate good, what our immediate profit is and we just cannot see past it. The frustration and / or pain and / or anger neutralizes our ability to see above or beyond the immediate and see that what we are really looking for, the answer to the question "What is our supreme good?" (And where the hell is it hiding?) In situations of frustration and / or pain and / or anger, the long-term, our growth and the other / collective is the last thing we are concerned about. But, if we can stop for a moment, step out of the boundaries of our immediate good and ask: "What is our supreme good? That could bring us far more quickly, to accept the situation, to achieve greater calm, a spiritual perspective and later on to change our course of action and achieve true change.

## Is it real or am I imagining it?

Another effect of the neutralization of our ability to look at the situation from above / from the side in order to see the situation (due to the frustration, pain or anger) is an additional reason for why it is so difficult for us to advance and to extract ourselves from certain painful situations . It is the fact that in these situations *the reality that we experience and receive is not an objective reality but our own personal interpretation that we bring to these situations.* This interpretation of events is based both on our past experience and our "character" and it can sometimes interfere with our ability to see things as they truly are. That is why if two people hear the same story from a third person, one will treat it as the end of the world or spend all day thinking about it whereas the other will nod and move on as if nothing had happened. For example, when we catch someone lying about something work-related, a small lie, but this lie drives us nuts. Our colleague, when in the same situation reacts by saying, "What a liar he is" but in the same breath adds "But what do I care?" and goes on to the next e-mail. We are driven nuts by the lie because we are oversensitive to lies (either because we have been lied to too much in our past or else because we constantly lie to others, or to ourselves, without being aware of it).

A few additional examples for illustration purposes:

- Our boss bumps into us in the hallway and casually mentions he would like to meet with us. We are hysterical and anxious about the meeting. We are sure he is about to fire us since we have really been slacking off lately and have been arriving late to work. Perhaps we even bad-mouthed him a few times behind his back and he found out about it. However, what he really wants to do is to consult with us regarding the development of a given product, offer us a promotion or ask us something personal in a field he knows we are knowledgeable.

- A female friend makes a casual remark about our outfit, saying it looks odd or unusual. We enter an emotional maelstrom and bitterness along the lines of "Who the hell does she think she is to tell us anything about the way we dress? Look at how she looks!" This is because we are simply unable to absorb and contain any type of external criticism having passed a critical threshold of accumulated criticism over too many years.

- Our spouse mentions that he or she has a really hard time living in a mess. This remark slams into our weak spots of frustration and berating ourselves, opening up a Pandora's Box of internal pain -- even though our spouse intended no complaint or criticism towards us.

- Our child is going to a sleepover party at a friend. We cannot sleep at night; we are so filled with anxieties since we are so used to think of all the terrible things that can happen in any given situation and at any given moment.

- Something goes missing and we cannot find it. We are immediately sure that "The world is full of thieves" and "Things are always being stolen here" because we have previously experienced theft of items. (Of course, the next day we find out that we have simply placed the item elsewhere or hidden it.)

- Suspicious signs lead us to suspect our spouse of cheating on us since we have suffered infidelity in the past and we are super sensitive to the situation -- when he was actually planning a surprise party.

In summary, we can, under certain conditions, be oversensitive (due to our past and our character), be driven by this negative emotion and be led to an interpretation of the situation that can cloud reality or blind us to its truth. It is recommended that we remember that there is always another way to look at things (which is why friends sometimes give us another angle on situations) and that our way might be slanted and therefore not objective. This is not because something is screwed up or wrong with us but because the mechanism of "oversensitive-interpretation-reality-twisting" exists in most human beings in various intensities and hues. That is simply the way we are made.

## *So what do we actually get out of this?*

What is the silver lining we are hunting for? Where is the good hiding within the evil that we experience or feel stuck in? What are we illuminating with our torch? Thus, this unseen benefit embodies all those things that we get from this situation and all of the things we learn from the situation. In other words, all of the things that ultimately benefit us in this situation (and we are not, of course, talking about any sort of material-financial profit). So what can get from harsh, painful and even cruel situations or events? We can get things that we are better aware of as well as things that we are not necessarily aware of (and which we often require considerable honesty and courage to admit). These include: Control of the situation, existential security, a feeling of belonging, love (either of self or the other), a rise in our self-value, calm or serenity, change or alteration, a platform or an opportunity for self-expression, discovery and connection to the destination, knowledge and insights or even abilities (physical or metaphysical), of which we were not aware.

*A few examples for illustration purposes:*
*Addictions*: An addiction is a difficult and complex situation that can even lead to the loss of your life (depending particularly on the type and amounts of the addictive substance but not only). Moreover, an addicted individual is an individual who is fleeing pain. He dulls it in order avoid suffering from whatever it is he is running from and, along the way, without meaning to, he creates a different type of pain, both to himself

and to his environment. However, this is not something he can really control. A dulling of pain is what he gets out of the situation and that is his profit from it. In certain cases, this experience might even be acquiring knowledge that will be useful in the future such as in the case of drug addicts who are rehabilitated and learn how to become rehab instructors. Their knowledge, born out of their own personal experience, makes them excellent instructors and supporters of their charges who also know exactly what the person undergoing withdrawal whom they are supporting / instructing is going through and enables them to bring true compassion born of empathy into the situation. The individual undergoing rehabilitation knows that they are not merely speaking hollow words to him but are speaking from their heart and from their own experience. This is a very powerful thing.

Well, what about the spouse of the addict? What does he or she get out of this situation? Seemingly, they are merely suffering, right? After all, it cannot be simple to live with an addict. This has many implications on many levels (relationship / sexual / financial / family / quality of life / shame). No matter how difficult this may sound, *an individual who is in a relationship with an addicted person also derives some type of profit from the situation*:

- Maybe it won't be easy for him when his spouse or significant other weans himself from his addiction because he will then become a completely different person?

- Perhaps he is used to the situation and is afraid of change?

- Perhaps he needs to take care of someone else?

- Perhaps he feels better about himself because there is someone in a worse situation than he is?

- Perhaps this is how he can control the situation and this control instills him with confidence?

- Alternatively, maybe this is the only way he feels needed, when someone desperately needs his help?

**The death of a loved one:** This is a difficult situation where we are forced to say farewell to a loved one and often experience great pain and heartbreak. Nonetheless, even in this extreme and difficult condition, there is always something we can take with us, learn or profit from including:

- Lessons about how to behave and not to behave.

- What is truly important in life.

- A lesson in courage or faith.

- Another opening of the heart.

- Understanding how important it is to speak about things and to work them out.

- A vast lesson in forgiveness (particularly when you are with a person on his deathbed).

- A wake-up call for how important life truly is.

- The value of life / the gift called life.

- Proportions.

- Getting a push to do something we have been avoiding to do because suddenly you understand that in any given moment one can die in a car accident or fall down the stairs.

**A severe disease**: Another difficult situation which, on the one hand, contains a great deal of suffering and pain, both physical and psychological, and, on the other hand, that very same disease has a high potential for benefits:

- Attention that we may be secretly yearning for.

- A relief and reprieve from many distasteful commitments or effort we do not really want to invest.

- Receiving a doctor's approval to whine and complain and perhaps even get some slack from those near from us because we are sick and miserable.

In addition, a severe disease is an incredible opportunity for change and development in many fields and on many levels in life:

- In our lifestyle, (a chance to undertake a long-awaited change in our diet and reduce the level of stress in our life).

- A change in the attitude of the environment to us and our attitude towards ourselves.

- Learning self-love and daring to listen to ourselves (sometimes for the first time in our lives)

- Learning to recognize our own value (both our own recognition and that of our environment).

- Accepting the courage to express the deepest depths of our hearts.

All of these changes lead to greater connection to the self which is why many call their disease "my gift." For them, it was an incredible chance to change whatever was not supporting their body or their soul, something that would never have occurred under any other circumstances. This severe disease also served as a platform and motivating force for that long-desired change. It is not difficult to find people who sat down in a wheelchair because of a fatal accident or a disease that say the same thing -- that the accident or wheelchair is the best thing that ever happened to them because that is how they discovered in themselves strengths and capabilities which they never would have drawn upon had it not been for that seemingly terrible disability which had been forced upon them and which they never wanted. This is a matter of choice, of course. What do we choose to focus upon, the good or the evil? Where do we choose to turn our attention? At the terrible evil, the great and the apparent? Alternatively, do we choose to focus on the good, even if it is tiny and perhaps still hidden and requires more to investigate and find? This is all a matter of choice. *Our subjective choice in a wider objective perspective.*

So where is the silver lining in the cloud hiding? Are we prepared to start looking for it? Are we ready to shine the "good torch" (which is essentially joyful and positive) even on hard and extreme situations as well as upon situations of lesser pain and suffering so that we might find in both types of situations our supreme good, the objectivity and the two things which we stand to gain from them -- acceptance (a response to hidden or apparent need or else the development of desired or neglected character traits) and learning (important lessons, knowledge or new capabilities)? If we succeed in finding all of these "treasures," this will lead to growth. Our growth.

## Summary of the first question -- where is the silver lining in the cloud?

- When we are in pain, angry or suffering, we are on "the dark side of the moon" and we do not feel like leaving it or trying harder just in order to see the "light" on the other side.

- The positive and joyful question "Where is the silver lining in the cloud?" is based on the assumption that every situation or event contains something good. This question forces us to be positive and to leave the negativity to which we are accustomed, forcing us to find our growth potential.

- Our supreme good is our "big picture" good that deals with the long-range and not the short, that deals with our growth and our development and that leaves the boundaries of the "me" entering into the territory of the "we."

- Our supreme good is quite often the exact opposite of our immediate good and this is frustrating and annoying, particularly when it is painful or when it is hard and we want it to just end and end now.

- The reality that we experience and perceive is not an objective reality but our personal-emotional interpretation that is based on our experience and character and it can blur reality or blind our eyes.

- The "oversensitive- biased interpretation- bent reality" mechanism exists in most human beings in various intensities and shapes. It is not that we are the only ones who are screwed up; it is simply part of the human condition.

- The silver lining which we seek in the most difficult situations embodies our supreme good, objectivity and the two types of benefits that hard situations provide us with: Things we receive (a response to hidden or apparent needs, the development of desired or neglected character traits) and what we learn (important lessons, knowledge and experience or new capabilities).

## 2 Why Did We Create this Situation?

The second question of the trilogy is much more challenging than the first since it requires that we take an additional step, a step that is not necessarily easy for us to take when we are in a difficult place, when we feel pain and when we experience suffering. That step is taking personal responsibility for our situation. Given the emotional complexity of the challenge and in order to receive precise, honest and practical answers that will lead us down the path that is right for us and get us out of the dead end we are in with maximal efficiency. It is recommended we call upon self-compassion and use no berating of ourselves in our inquiry. *We are not guilty and we are not looking for a guilty party. We are seeking the higher reasons and the solutions to them.* We are efficient. The second question needs to be split into two parts which are both separate and interlinked: *The first part deals with the creation of the situation (how reality forms) and the second part deals with the why (the world of lower and higher causes behind creation).*

## *How does reality form?*

Who among us has not heard the sentences "thought creates reality" or "spirit effects matter?" To some of us this is new age prattle at best or spiritualist nonsense at worst. However, the single distilled essence at the base of these two sentences is what is running our lives, both consciously and unconsciously. If we wish to achieve greater control of the situation, greater spiritual perspective as well as more serenity in our lives, it is better that we put aside our initial resistance, should such exist and see what is the true basis of these sentences, what they are all about and whether they have any grounding in reality.

*The physical level* – we will start with the scientific facts because it is easier for some us to open up our hearts and ears when something has scientific backing. Our ego, which safeguards us from being hurt or disappointed, will also receive the dosage of logic and common sense that it so urgently requires and then there is a chance that it will not disturb us in the future.

The consciousness of researchers has repeatedly been shown to affect the results of experiments[13] in subatomic particles.

---

13      Those of us who are not physicists and wish to understand how consciousness changes the physical properties of matter are invited to watch the movie of Dr. Quantum, a simple to understand animation movie is intended for the general public about the two aperture experiment. (A well-known experiment from the world of Quantum Physics and one of the great mysteries of this world and its consequences)www.youtube.com/watch?v=yS3DXQ9jY04.

In quantum physics this phenomenon is known as the "Observer Effect." (A term from the world of science which describes the way in which an observer who is watching and measuring a given phenomenon might change the dynamic he is observing.) Another relevant term from the world of social sciences is the "*observer bias.*" This term describes an error in the experiment which occurs when the observers, frequently the researchers, overemphasize the behavior or outcome they expect to receive and do not even observe those behaviors and outcomes that they do not expect. This is a well-known and significant phenomenon which is why medical research experiments try to overcome this "problem" by performing a "double blinded" experiment in which both the researcher and the subject of the experiment are not aware of the expected outcome as they are not aware of which experimental group (such as the control group which receives a placebo) they had been assigned to.

In other words, where human consciousness is involved, it has direct impact on matter. Our metaphysical consciousness affects the physical. The metaphysical consciousness can be identified with our thoughts, our beliefs, our conclusions and our desires, both conscious and unconscious. Spirit does indeed affect matter and the material reality in which we live. *What we believe and what we think will happen truly impacts what actually happens. The energy flows wherever we focus our consciousness.*

*The biological-physical level* – "The placebo effect" (an improvement in the medical conditioning of an individual who received an inactive substance that he thought was medication) and the "nucebo effect" (a negative development in the condition of an individual who was given a negative diagnosis or just heard a discouraging sentence from a health professional.) are well known scientific phenomenon. Both are proof of the fact that the human body responds, on the biological-chemical level in accordance to the beliefs of the individual. It is highly recommended that you read Bruce Lipton's, "The Biology of Belief" which explains in simple and clear language, (with illustrations and examples from dozens of supporting scientific studies), how beliefs impact our biology and how our genes are activated and regulated by our environment – the food we ingest, the thoughts we think about ourselves, our behavior and our lifestyle. If we believe that we will develop a given disease just because everyone in our family is ill with it, we truly will fall victim to it. If the doctor whom we implicitly believe and who enjoys our blind trust tells us that our chances of overcoming the disease are small, then our body will respond accordingly and all of our systems will be activated and respond accordingly. If, on the other hand, that physician tells us that we will surely overcome the disease -- then that is what will happen on the physiological level. People have been shown to throw up and lose their hair when they were told they were receiving a chemotherapeutic pill when in practice they were receiving a pill with inactive materials. In other words, their body was behaving in accordance to what they believed and expected regardless of the actual treatment they received. It has furthermore been found that people with a strong social network were only half as likely to develop heart conditions in comparison to lonely people, that optimist people were 77% less likely to develop heart diseases than pessimistic people and that happy people lived 7-10 years longer than sad people.[14] *Our consciousness creates a physiological reality that matches whatever we believe in.*

*On the psychological-soul level* -- Our soul is composed of thoughts and emotions. We have already seen in the chapter dealing with exchanging berating oneself with self-compassion what destructive consequences words have on our emotions, on our behavior and our character. We have also seen how the conclusions we made as a result of difficult and painful events in our life have developed into beliefs and self-perceptions using these neural pathways in our brain and which became our "absolute truth" which runs us and through which we perceive reality. In other words, our soul, through our responses and our behavior, creates a certain reality that matches these thoughts and these emotions. We have thousands of thoughts every day (on a very wide spectrum of depth and importance) and each thought has an emotion which matches it. (If, for example, we think "I hate this man," we will automatically feel an emotion of hatred which might even be associated with a physical response such as clenched

---

14     A movie clip that explains and illustrates this simply is "Ted Talk" of Dr. Lissa Rankin, "Scientific Proof that We Can Heal Ourselves." Is there scientific proof we can heal ourselves? Lissa Rankin, M.D., www.youtube.com/watch?v=LWQfe__fNbs&t=409s

muscles, redness in the faface or rapid breathing). These are all broadcast out into the world. It can be said that we are like a powerful broadcast tower that is constantly operating and that each one of us has his own personal frequency that is being broadcast out into the world and draws to it situations, people and events that respond to this frequency.

An extreme example that illustrates this very well is that of a battered woman. No woman wishes to be beaten, to be abused and to have pain inflicted on her repeatedly or all the other terrible things that such a woman needs to deal with. Nonetheless, it often seems that battered women show a pattern of repeatedly finding themselves with violent men. Even when a battered woman finds the strength to break away and flee such a destructive relationship, she can easily find herself in another violent and destructive relationship. Why is this? After all, she does not desire to be beaten and abused; she does not wish this for herself, does she? Nonetheless, if we should examine the belief system of this woman, some of them, if not most, will be subconscious. We will find such beliefs as "I deserve to be beaten" and / or "I don't deserve any better" and / or "Who will respect me? And / or "who will even want me?" The source of these beliefs is in her personal history. This personal history frequently includes verbal and physical violence, humiliation, lack of respect and a shaky and hurtful relationship model. In other words, the woman broadcasts subconsciously and inadvertently, beliefs such as "I deserve to be beaten" and the men who approach her are those who match this frequency (*like attracts like*). It is her subconscious beliefs that form a difficult and cruel reality.

It is important to note that *it is not the fault of the battered woman. She is not guilty of anything and she never wished to be beaten.* However, she was broadcasting this outwards, even if subconsciously, and that is why it is so important to develop awareness of both the obvious layers of our soul and its hidden layers as well.

## It is not really that simple…

We have seen that we create our reality on several levels – physical, biological and psychological -- and that we are a type of broadcast tower that is constantly broadcasting out to the world. So why can't we successfully create what we truly desire? Why aren't any of us magicians that can conjure into existence anything our heart desires? Why can't we summon into our life the yacht or the billion dollars in the bank which will set us up for life or the perfect body we fantasize about or the significant other we so desire?

*The first reason* – absence of faith. We do not really believe we create our reality. Our logic and common sense rule it out. Even if we should hear a thousand stories of individuals who created a certain reality or called something into their lives (and saw it appear), some part of us will still say that that cannot happen, not to us, and that only others are so fortunate -- we do not have a chance at winning the jackpot. Why are we so faithless? Firstly, most of us are fundamentally negative, remember? Our automatic response is always to say no. Secondly, most of us live in the past (or are afraid of the future) and we let it dictate the shape of our present – we did not succeed in the past so there is no reason for us to succeed now. Thirdly, our ego has a defensive mechanism that guards us from being disappointed and hurt again, as in the past, which is why it raises very logical claims such as "It is better not to even get into it." "This is just disappointment / chicanery / someone here is trying to make money off of us." "We already know better than to believe this nonsense."

Classic examples of this absence of faith can be seen in attempts to summon parking. Many people have read in the book "The Secret" (or watched the movie), that parking can be summoned at any place and at any time, right? However, many of us have tried and failed. Why? Because you cannot summon parking (truly imagining that sweet parking spot just waiting for us to pull in) while you say / think / believe that "There is no way to find parking at these hours" or "This street never has any parking." The two do not go together and the one nullifies the other.

*The second reason – the rule of the subconscious.* Karl Jung summed it up splendidly when he said: "*Until you transform your subconscious into your conscious, it will run your life and you will call it fate.*" Our conscious only controls a small fraction of our essence. (On the neurological level, the brain processes hundreds of *billions* of data points a second and we are conscious of only 2,000 of them.) The subconscious is our true ruler. It determines what we say, what we feel, what we decide, how we respond and how we act under certain situations and in front of certain people. The subconscious contains all of the conclusions we have made from the events of our life and all of the beliefs that were formed by these conclusions. If we take, for example, a man who has both a conscious belief system (of which he is aware and about which he consciously thinks) which includes such thoughts as: "Nothing ever works out for me." "I keep on failing all the time." "The world is full of thieves." as well as other limited, but subconscious belief systems that contain such beliefs as: "Only others enjoy wealth and plenty." "I have nothing to contribute to anyone." or else "I don't deserve to win / enjoy / receive." If that same man decides to summon into his life glamorous and expensive sports cars, he can drop to his knees and imagine it until steam comes out of his ears five times a day, every day, how he will drive in the car and how his hair will wave in the wind and how the hottest girl he knows will be sitting next to him but that sports car will not show up and neither will the hot girl because his subconscious has too much power. It is the subconscious that decides and determines and if that subconscious believes that a man does not deserve the good fortune he desires then that good fortune simply will not arrive. Furthermore, that man can dream / imagine, summon the luxurious sports car ten times a day but rest assured that his subconscious mind, if not his conscious mind, will be running through thoughts and fears of want and poverty 300 times a day ("I will never get out of debt." "I have no money, I am barely surviving." "There are no jobs to be found." "Life is hard.") Take a wild guess – which thoughts will dominate the other in the real world? The good news is that one can discover and reach these limiting beliefs (in other words these highways in our brain), meet them, answer them and at the same time create new, alternate, beliefs.

*The third reason – the existence of important reasons.* Every one of us has a certain script for his life and every one of us has his destiny (which embodies the gift and uniqueness he brings to the world). If something we really want is not in the script and is not part of our destiny, then it will not be fulfilled no matter how hard we imagine it and how many efforts and actions we undertake.

There are supreme reasons for everything and they all include the same script and the same destination. Few of us know from birth what we are here to do and what type of occupation will makes us get up in the morning happy and with a profound sense of satisfaction (and even that can be temporary and only up to a certain point in life). Most of us do not know and this is a very frustrating situation. That is why we need the connection to the highest level of ourselves, to the spirit, to the part within us that does know what is the way we are meant to travel in this life and can help us discover what is right and possible for us at this specific point in time. This also requires patience, a great deal of patience, which cannot be bought in any store.

## *Why does the Zebra wear striped pajamas?*

The existence of these important reasons is the connection point between the second part of the question, "Why did we create this situation?" which dealt with the creation of this situation (how the reality is formed), to this part, which deals with the 'why" of the situation, with the world of lower and higher reasons behind the creation of the situation. Before we expand upon the "'why" and see how it can be found, we will familiarize ourselves with another axiom that will aid us in this search – *"The outer world is a reflection of the inner word." In other words, everything that occurs in the external reality of our lives is a reflection of the reality within us.* The events, situations and people whom we face at any given point in time, reflect, represent and are directed at the inner aspects within us that require solutions, some of which are distressed and are ripe at that specific point in time to rise into awareness and be cured (if they were not, then they would not have shown up in our lives at that point in time). For example, if we are in a situation where we are being dismissed or disparaged, *this aspect is already part of us, interwoven as a narrative in our personal biography -- and it is seeking a response, healing or release.* The first stage is acknowledging this aspect, recognizing that it is there. If we recognize that we are being lied to in a number of situations, then there are grounds to reflect where else in our lives we have had to face lies (whether we have been lied to by others, lied to others or lied to ourselves). Reflection should be based on an understanding that these instances of lying are filled with pain and suffering and that it is time to bring that pain and suffering to the surface and to let it go. The outer lie is signaling to us as if it were realizing a formal distress call: "Mayday, Mayday, Mayday," that there is an inner lie that must be dealt with. *The external grappling with the outer lie is an invitation to dive into our inner depths and provide help and healing to the place of inner pain.*

When we deal with the why and seek the reasons for that why, it is worth bearing in mind that reasons include both the primary and the supreme reasons (deriving from the spirit within us), which contains our life script and our destination, as well as the world of lower, earthly reasons (the world of the body -- soul) which contains our thoughts and feelings, both conscious and subconscious.

For the most part, we will not know at any given moment what these higher reasons are or even what the lower, subconscious reasons are. However, we can certainly take action to reveal or expose them so that they might help us answer the question, "Why did we create this situation?" by:

1. *Calming down the system* (meditation, a nature walk, yoga, garden work…), listening to the spirit, that same spirit which whispers rather than shouts. We should define our intention of receiving information and then see what, if any, information comes. We are not always ready or ripe to get the answers that we seek.

2. *Stretching out our antennas and begin seeking out the signs the spirit is scattering for us to find* -- In the first chapter, the one dealing with the three-part nature of man, we saw that the spirit's style of communication is extremely sophisticated and not necessarily verbal. The answers to the questions we asked can be found in any component of the environment of our reality -- a headline in the newspaper, a song on the radio,

a coincidental conversation on the street / standing in line / riding the bus, a message on a street sign, an insight from a movie film / a TV series and so on.

3. *Identifying and acknowledging supportive probabilities and coincidences* -- As mentioned previously, our sublime good is the basis of our existence and we therefore occasionally receive (but do not always recognize) "slight nudges" from life that push us forward. These nudges appear in the shape of events, situations or people which are exactly what we needed at that moment of our lives -- we met the exactly right person or situation we needed to move us forward, to help us, to support us, to assist us or to explain to us and teach us -- the right person at the right time. Sometimes this is a truly "insane" coincidence of which we would likely say "What are the odds of this happening?" Still, our friend Albert Einstein put it well: *"Coincidences are simply God's way of remaining anonymous."*

## Questions, questions, questions. So many questions....

Below are a list of directed questions that can help us locate that "why?" and from that starting point insert the required changes into our lives. Remember, the goal is not to assign guilt but to find solutions. Let us not forget to look at things through the glasses of self-compassion:

**What are we missing?** Let us put aside the "one million dollar" answer that 99.99% of the people would do very well with a million dollars in the bank, thank you very much. Let us instead consider whether there is any personality trait which we would like to adopt (such as courage, generosity, sensitivity, acceptance, flexibility, ability to express ourselves, ability to relax and take things easy, openness to new experiences…). Perhaps we are missing the ability to openly communicate with someone in our life (a parent, a spouse, a sibling, a child, a colleague, a friend) and perhaps we would like to adopt a certain value (such as self-respect or being able to respect the other, fairness, belonging, authenticity, compassion, stability, existential security…).

**What is stuck?** The answer to the question "Where are we stuck?" also includes the question, "What is not flowing smoothly in our lives without us noticing?" (in the family, in our career, in our relationships or in our self-perception)? And also, "What is not progressing at all or not progressing sufficiently and at the proper pace for me?" Are we, ourselves, holding up a given process? Alternatively, are we perhaps being held up by external forces?

**What are we not fulfilling?** Have we had an old childhood dream or any dream which we have never been able to realize, that has been pushed aside or hidden away because of social or family pressure such as: "Study for a respectable profession." "A personal coach / social worker doesn't make any money." "Only you can take the helm of the family business." "Thousands of people want to succeed in this field, your chances are non-existent, go for something safe." "It is very dangerous out there." "What will the neighbors say? Don't shame us." "At your age you need to start planning for your retirement." Or "Where do you come up with the nonsense in your head?" It could be that the feeling of being stuck we experience in the field of our activity is meant to lead us back onto the track which we were supposed to follow in the first place, the true aim for which our soul yearned, which brought out the best of us with ease and with joy and which took our breath away each time anew. Alternatively, perhaps this feeling of being stuck is meant to motivate us to fulfill our destiny, personal or social. The world is filled with people who found their true destiny after harsh and challenging events. It is worthwhile to ask these questions and to let them echo in our minds and hearts for a while.

**What is striving to get out?** Which aspects of our soul, deep within, wish to receive attention or are seeking relief and healing? We walk on the face of this earth like sacks stuffed with emotional waste. This waste is made up of pain (both old and new), stress, traumatic events, fears and anxieties, anger and rage (both hidden and apparent), shame, guilt and a great deal of berating oneself and even hatred -- every one of us with his own composition and dosages of this emotional waste. Those aspects of our soul which have experienced these harsh emotions over many years and still experience them in the present -- even if decades have gone by since the events themselves took place -- are seeking attention and relief. They are seeking release and healing. The feeling of being stuck we feel in the present serves as a sort of traffic sign directing us towards those painful places that want to release the pain, that want to stop hurting already. Those of us who are afraid to touch old pains again can be comforted by the fact that these pains are internal and would not have gone anywhere if they had not risen to the surface, would not have risen up in the form of these blockages and these situations had we not been ready and ripe to confront them and to deal with them. We must trust creation and its precision and rely on the principle that things turn out as they do for our supreme good. Most of all, we must have faith in ourselves and our ability to deal with our internal aches and pains.

***What does this situation reflect for us?*** Often, we cannot see something directly because we are not aware of it or because it is too hard, too dim, too painful, too embarrassing or too humiliating, too frightening or too scary. That is why the spirit will walk the extra mile towards us and reflect to us that aspect within ourselves that is seeking attention / help / recognition / healing, through people and situations in our reality. Considerable honesty is required to be able to see this reflection which will mostly deal with our less attractive, to put it mildly, parts. Those of us who are parents can see it quite easily in their children. They have qualities or behaviors that remind us of ourselves at their age -- or even as adults. However, it is not merely our children who reflect our internal aspects for us, it is everyone who surrounds us who reflects these things, some of them positive and some negative, some things we wish to acquire and some things that we would love to shed. However, we must be capable of recognizing the reflections and the situations in which reflections exist in order to fully fulfill the potential in this situation.

*The key for successful identification of these reflections is very simple -- whatever I see on the outside must also exist within me at one level or another. The hue might be somewhat different but it is most certainly there, else I would not be confronting it in the external world.* The well-known aphorism, "The pot calling the kettle black" is a type of "twin" of this reflection. Whatever we criticize, reject, judge and badmouth in others, is part of us as well. If, for example, we find ourselves judging a certain parent from our child's class, repeatedly telling ourselves that he is not investing sufficiently time and attention in his child or that he does not care what happens with his child, this is the place to be honest with ourselves and see where and when we behave in this manner with our own child. Something in the behavior we are criticizing or judging must be part of us as well else we would not be so judgmental regarding this issue. It is simply much easier for us to see this in the other rather than in ourselves.

## A reflection, exercise and internalization stop

*The reflection exercise (also known as the mirror method), is one of the greatest gifts we can grant ourselves as it maps the reflections in our life. Our reflections are all of the people in our life, near and far alike, who have come to teach us something about ourselves. They do so by reflecting to us, by their* behavior, something that is part of us as well. *The rule is – whatever irritates us, reflects us. Whatever angers us, reflects us.* The simplest way to map out the reflections in our life is to:

1. To list all of the people who irritate us.

2. To check and write down what is the *specific thing* with each and every one of them which pisses us off / irritates us / angers us / unbalances us / drives us nuts. It is best if you can distill whatever that individual "does to us" to one or two words. For example: He humiliates us, he lies to us, he disrespects us, he doesn't listen to us, he shames us, he only thinks of himself, he is uncaring, he is uncivilized in his behavior, he frightens us, he is neglectful, he is always angry / irritated / grumpy / critical of others.

3. *Search within.* After we go through this distillation process and arrive at an understanding of the specific irritation, for example, "He always lies," we need to find how this quality is reflected within us. This can be *in the present* – do we constantly lie to others or ourselves in some way or another (even without noticing)? Or perhaps this pain is *in our past* -- when in our life, even in childhood, have we encountered a lie (either by lying ourselves or being lied to) in such a way that we were hurt and pained? How is the emotional memory of that pain still alive and beating inside us? *Are both true?*

> Have we perhaps been lied to in the past (either once or on an ongoing basis) and we therefore lie to others or to ourselves, in the present?
>
> Yes, the people who anger us the most and irritate us the most, are precisely the greatest mirrors in our lives, those who are giving us the greatest favor (in the big picture), those who lead us to our greatest growth.

If we summarize all of the questions we asked here in order to help us answer the question, "Why have we created this situation?" then it seems that they all lead to a place where we understand that a true change is needed in our lives -- whether on the personal, professional, family, relationship or several or all of the above. As soon as we understand the why (the lower and supreme reasons), it is much easier for us to work towards making changes in our lives out of a place of acceptance, compassion and a deep desire for growth, rather than conflict or self-hate.

## Summarizing the second question-- why did we create this situation?

- We are required to assume responsibility for the situation but we are neither guilty nor seeking those at fault. What we are seeking are the lower and supreme reasons for this situation whose identification will lead us to undertake the desired change.

- On the one hand, we create the reality we live in on

*several levels.* The physical level (consciousness affects the matter particles and changes it), on the physiological level (the body responds biologically in accordance to what man believes) and the psychological level (the soul creates a reality which matches its thought and emotions).

- On the other hand, we cannot truly create everything we might desire due to lack of faith (we are essentially negative, living in the past, defense mechanism), ruled by our subconscious (it is the part of our mind really running our lives) and the existence of supreme reasons (whatever is not part of our life's script and which is not part of our destiny will not come to pass).

- In order to discover the subconscious supreme and lower reasons, it is recommended:

  1. To *calm down* the system.
  2. To extend our antennas and seek the signs.
  3. To identify and acknowledge *supportive probabilities and coincidences.*

- "The external world is a reflection of the inner world" – the outer reality of our lives is a reflection of the inner reality within us (internal aspects in our lives that are seeking a response).

- Guiding questions which might help us discover the "*Why?*"

- *What are we missing?* Personal qualities, communication skills, a certain value.

- *What is obstructed?* What is not flowing, what is not progressing sufficiently or at all, are we being stalled or are we stalling?

- *What are we not fulfilling?* A childhood dream, an un-realized dream, a personal or social role you are meant to fulfill.

- *What is seeking release?* What aspects of our soul are seeking attention, relief and healing? The obstructions as traffic signs that are pointing us at painful places that are ripe to release the pain.

- *What does the situation reflect for us?* The thing within us that is crying out for help, attention and recognition or healing is reflected to us through various situations and people in our reality. The key for identification – whatever you see in the outer world exists in the inner world as well.

- *Our reflections* – the people in our lives teach us about ourselves by reflecting to us something that is within us. The rule of the thumb is – *whoever is irritating and angering us, is reflecting for us.*

- Understanding the "Why?" (The lower reasons, conscious and subconscious, and the supreme reasons), *eases the introduction of the desired changes* in our lives from a place of acceptance, compassion and a deep desire for growth, rather from a place of conflict or self-hate.

The Three Trilogy questions
# 3 What Can We Change?

**(in thought, emotion and actions)**

We have arrived at the practical question, the question that takes the theoretical insights that answering the first two questions provided us with and brings them down to earth, into the reality of our material lives, into the everyday life that includes the actions we perform, the emotions we feel and the thoughts we think. Our reality, after all, is made up of what we think (our thoughts accompanied by emotions), what we say and what we do. If we want to change this reality, we need to change ourselves; we need to change and this both scares us and feels a little unfair because why should we be the ones to change rather than everyone else?

We have already seen in the chapter dealing with the premise of the disguised opportunities how much we are threatened and scared by the word change and how much we hate and are afraid of changes, scared of the unknown, hate being uncertain (discomforted, shaken, stressed out and threatened). That is why we prefer to stick to the known and the familiar. That is why we prefer to stay where we have greater control of the situation -- even if it is no great catch, to put it mildly. This is why we stick to an unfulfilling job, a tyrant boss, a hated profession, boring friends, an unsupportive spouse, an environment we are not comfortable with or various addictions that are pleasant and comfort us on the short-term but are damaging to us on the long-term.

Furthermore, we have seen why it is so difficult for us to change our beliefs and our habits. We have seen how repeating the same behaviors (again and again and again) creates in our brain, on the physiological level, a highway onto which we automatically turn. These automatic paths of least resistance become what we think of as "our character" which is made up of these very same habits: A habit of responding in a certain way, a habit of behaving in a certain way, a habit of thinking in a certain way or a habit of speaking in a certain way.

In the previous chapter we have also seen why we are the ones who need to change and not everyone else. We have seen that the exterior world is in fact a reflection of our inner world and that external reality is a reflection of our inner reality. In particular, it is a reflection of internal aspects within us that are seeking attention and resolution. Some of these aspects are in a state of anxiety (the situation / obstruction that we feel is their official signal of distress, the "Mayday, Mayday" they are broadcasting) which is now ready to rise up into our awareness and receive the healing on that aching spot -- even if the pain is old. Diving into these inner depths in order to provide the necessary aid is what will trigger the necessary change. This is what will make us change.

## *It all begins and ends with the will to change*

To summarize, we want to change and to be changed because we are obstructed and because we realize that if do not change we will stay stuck in the same situation until it deteriorates further. At some point, something new will happen and we will get a little push from life in the form of conditions, events and situations that will force us to stop and reflect in order to help us and shift us from the place where we were stuck, in order to help us to continue to learn and grow. Yes, we might perceive this road as cruel, particularly if we lack a supreme spiritual perspective. But, if we want to change the reality of our lives or a specific situation in which we are stuck, then we need to assume responsibility for this situation, both for creating it (the understanding that we create the reality of our own lives, sometimes without being aware of it) and for undertaking the specific actions leading to moving past this situation, to getting unstuck.

Since change is both frightening (fear of the unknown and fear of pain) and difficult (the triumph of our habits) and is perceived by us sometimes as being unfair ("Somebody external is making us feel badly – he / she / they / it need to change!) Actually making change happen is difficult. It is so difficult that we feel that this is "impossible." The keyword here is will. We need to want to change. When Martin Luther King said that he had a dream that "one day this nation will rise up and live out the true meaning of its creed: "We hold these truths to be self-evident, that all men are created equal," that "my four little children will one day live in a nation where they will not be judged by the color of their skin but by the content of their character." When he spoke, these words seemed completely unrealistic and un-implementable, about as unrealistic as the intention of Gandhi to bring about the non-violent end of British imperial rule over India or our modern-day dream of peace in the Middle East. Like a fairytale. What made these dreams come true was will for change of these great people and their followers. Absent this will for change, the Union Jack might still be flying over India and segregation might well have remained the law of the land in the South.

If we do have a will to change and truly will change to happen, then there is no point on dwelling upon it and talking is a waste of time. If we do not truly will it, then nothing will change and we will continue to suffer. If we don't really want to change, then we will never really manage to change and be changed. Successful change requires considerable emotional strength, persistence, perseverance, courage, the ability to get back up when you fall (and you will fall) and all sorts of other qualities that not all of us have when we take the first step of our journey. And yet, should we but will it, deep inside we will be able to face and meet every challenge along the road and get up when we stumble and fall as we walk the path to change because nothing is set in stone and unchangeable (as we have seen, even the structure of our brain and gene regulation are subject to change,) if we want to make change happen and are prepared to do something to make it happen.

## *The first stage is changing how we think...*

The first thing we need to change is how we perceive the situation we are stuck in and what we think about it. In the chapter dealing with berating oneself and self-compassion, we saw that the reality (as we experience and perceive it) is not truly objective. Rather, what we perceive are layers of personalized interpretation that we bring into every situation we experience. These interpretations are based both on our experience and on our "character" (and that character, of course, is formed by habits of thought and action -- neural highways, remember?). We have seen that this personal interpretation can interfere with our ability to see challenging situations as they truly are since throughout our life we have experienced criticism and / or humiliation and / or intimidation and / or injuries and / or pain and / or shame and / or guilt and some part within us believes that all of the not nice things people have told us are true or that whatever happened to us was well-deserved. Furthermore, the conclusions and beliefs formed by these events in the past, through the neural pathways in our brain, have become our "absolute truth" which governs and runs us and through which we perceive reality. So, since our perception of life and situation has such immense importance, the first thing we need to do is to change the way we think, to change how we perceive our situation.

## How do we implement this in practice?

*First, we must operate and perform out of full self-awareness which is essentially the ability to look at our actions and behavior from the side.* We must become spectators who observe our situation as an external event for the purpose of rational analysis of the situation after we finish watching it. We must, in fact, detach ourselves from the situation itself because *this separation will grant us the objectivity we seek.* This detachment is our tool to dim the personal and sometimes twisted interpretation which we described above. If, for example, what is obstructing us is a cruel boss in the workplace who treats us badly and perhaps even humiliates us, which makes us hate him, curse him all day and focus our thoughts on planning creative ways to end his current state of existence, then what we need to do is relate to this situation as if it were happening to a close friend and their boss. This is no longer about us; this is about our friend, his boss, his workplace, his obstruction and his events and situations. This detachment will help us think clearly.

*The second stage is assembling data.* We centralize all the data that we gathered from the first two questions: ("Where is the silver lining in the cloud?" and "Why have we created this situation?"). By this point, we already have valuable information which includes various lists: *A list of benefits –* what we are getting from this situation (attention to hidden or known needs or the development of desired or neglected character traits) and what we learn from it (important lessons, knowledge, experience or new capabilities), a list of supreme and unconscious lower reasons that led to the formation of the situation (What are we missing? What is obstructed? What aren't we fulfilling? What within us is seeking release? What within us is seeking attention and recognition?) *and a list of reflections* (What does this situation reflect for us? What aspects of our soul are demanding attention, relief and healing?)

We concentrate all of the data from the various lists into a single master chart, look at it and let the data speak for itself. We let the data within that list drop the necessary chips for the formation of the will to change. *The answers to these questions are, in and of themselves, the solution to the situation.* Suddenly, there is not mere desperation but also hope. Suddenly, the obstructions or other situations we experience are no longer "the most terrible thing that has ever happened to us." Suddenly, there is not merely a cloud but also a silver lining. Suddenly, this is hope amid the desperation, and clarity among the confusion. Suddenly, there is not just obstruction but also movement.

To get back to the example of the cruel boss who treats us cruelly and who humiliates us, this is the time and place to examine the reflection of this man in our lives:

- Why is he actually there?
- What is he trying to teach us about ourselves?
- Where is the cruelty and humiliation that is reflected

without representation within?

- Where in our past (throughout our life) have we been treated this way?

- Were we similarly hurt in the past (one-time, continuously or repetitively)?

- Are we, perhaps, behaving in a similar (though slightly different) manner in the present? Is this how we are behaving, without even noticing it, to someone else?

- Are we perhaps being cruel to ourselves?

- Do we somehow believe we do not deserve to be treated well?

- Do we have some sort of belief that only toughness or intimidation gets things done?

- Alternatively, perhaps some inner aspect of ourselves dismisses or constantly doubts every one of our achievements?

The answers to these questions are the basis for the next steps in our journey. If we still cannot find the answers, we are not being sufficiently honest and open with ourselves or are still not sufficiently detached from the situation. *This is a chance to ask a good friend or a person dear to our hearts, who we know wishes the best for us to help us with external reflection.* We will ask him to answer these questions concerning our situation and see what insights he can provide and what he thinks of the situation.

*The third stage is to write down a list of new perspectives.*

We make a new list of all of the new thoughts we want, are considering or can adopt. *These thoughts contain, in their base and in their essence, our spiritual perspective and supreme good which combines within it our development and our growth, our long-term perspective and the emergence from the boundaries of "me" towards "we."* Here are a few examples of new thoughts and perspectives that we might develop in regard to this cruel boss of ours:

- Thanks to our boss, we are, for the first time in our lives, learning more about ourselves and know ourselves better.

- Thanks to his cruelty, we are diving in and paying attention to the parts within us that have suffered and have been suffering for so many years. Thanks to him, we are finally healing ourselves.

- Thanks to his humiliating approach, we finally understand that we are no longer willing to be spoken to in this manner. No more!

- We can suddenly see that our boss is himself miserable because he has his own boss who is even more terrible, who terrorizes him all day. Our direct boss simply dumps all of his frustration on us because this is his way for dealing with his own difficulties. That may not justify his behavior but it does separate the quality of our work from the unjustified negative feedback we are receiving from him.

- Thanks to his cruel behavior, we have come to understand that we have no wish to stay in a workplace with such a deeply flawed organizational culture. We want to move on and get to a workplace with a more humane, embracing and caring organizational culture.

These thoughts are the basis and the foundations of the new consciousness which we want to adopt. It will always be our choice on what we choose to focus on: The cloud or the silver lining? The half-full or half-empty glass? The obstruction or the change?

## Then we change the way we feel...

After we have the list of new thoughts, it is time to get to work on our emotions. As we already know, *our emotions and thoughts are interwoven, affect and are affected by each other and so it is not enough to merely change what we think about the situation, it is also necessary to change what we feel about it.*

If we think love – we feel love.
If we think hate – we feel hate.

And the opposite is also true.

If we feel love – we will definitely think thoughts of love.
And if we feel hate – we will definitely think hateful thoughts.

*A reflection, practice and internalization stop*

The simplest and easiest way to understand the *meaning of the connection between our thoughts and emotions* is to sample specific words and the physical sensations that accompany these words. For example, say the following words out loud: Hatred, anger, fear, cheating, evil, cruelty or violence (each word separately and on its own) and to note how our body responds and which sensations arise (trembling, tense contractions, heavy breathing, rage, unease...). Conversely, the following words can also be said aloud: Love, compassion, joy, unconditional giving, harmony or laughter (each word separately and one at a time) and note how our body responds and what physical sensations arise (expansion, thrill, joy, glee, peace, calm...).

If, for example, we hate a given situation, we cannot develop the willpower to change it because the emotion of hate surrounds us and dominates us, twisting our thoughts, creating lack of clarity and focus, clouding our vision (blurring reality) and activating our ego which will seek to protect us at all costs, perhaps even by harming someone else. The broadcasting tower which is us will be broadcasting hate-filled frequencies outside and life will bring us other things, events and situations, that match this hatred frequency (in accordance with the principle "like attracts like") which will, in turn, fan the existing hatred even more. Just like oil on a fire, we will continue to hate more and more and, most of all, we will continue to suffer and remain stuck.

## How do we implement this in practice?

*The first stage is to recognize what emotion is operating in this case.* Is the emotion that accompanies this situation or obstruction an emotion of hate, fear, shame, anger or guilt? By identifying this emotion, *we are admitting to ourselves that we are feeling it.* We are putting it on the table, making it present and ceasing to ignore it.

*The second stage is to express a conscious wish to change this emotion.* We declare that we want and choose to cease hating, being angry or feeling guilty and thereby assume responsibility for changing the situation. We thereby declare to ourselves that we do not expect anyone else to change and that only internal change will lead to the desired external change. It is not that by expressing the wish to change that emotion it will immediately change or disappear. The path ahead is far longer than that. But this statement has its own strength and it, in turn, supports and assists the process.

*In the third stage, we locate channels through which these negative emotions can be cleaned out and drained away.* Merely draining this emotional waste outside of us (through psycho-logical-emotional, energetic or spiritual treatment, through the use of guided imagination, by putting things down in writing, by slamming a punching bag or even by screaming into a pillow) will lead to considerable relief. We will feel significantly lighter and less uptight and that will allow new emotions in because when you clear emotional space, room for something new to come in forms.

In the fourth stage we appreciate the opportunity because true appreciation (from the heart), leads to emotional change. A feeling of thankfulness is the most efficient, the most helpful and the most productive emotion and the one which most contributes to positive change. If we use the example of the cruel boss again: How much can we really continue to hate someone who eventually made us feel better (no matter how much he made us suffer before we began getting better), who led us to take a path of self-improvement and growth, who led us to reconnect to ourselves and who brought us to a place which is much better for us? At this stage, if we performed the necessary work on our thoughts, emotions and perspectives, if we have drained away the evil and understood where good is, the emotion of hate will rapidly shift to a feeling of appreciation -- appreciation of everything we achieved thanks to this individual -- even if he himself does not change and even if there is still no way to justify how he is behaving.

*And then, finally, we change what we do...*

After we are done changing how we think and feel, it is time to change how we act. This is the stage where we move from talk to action. This is the stage where we move from changes within to changes without. This is the stage where we move from thoughts and emotions to actions: What can we do differently? How can we behave differently? How can we respond differently? How can we speak differently?

*The inner change we have performed so far (in thought and in emotion) is what will enable us to perform the external change because there is no other way to make a change. The correct order is from within to without.* A change that is merely external does not change anything on the inside and therefore will not last long. It will collapse in the form of a return to the bad, old, automatic habits as soon as a new challenge or crisis emerges. At this stage, we already know that whatever crisis comes knocking at our door is, in fact, a type of opportunity in disguise which is here precisely in order to back up the change in the form of an action that will prove to ourselves and to the world that we have actually succeeded in changing. After all, we can talk about change forever, but what actually matters is the actions we take and their outcome in reality.

## How do we implement this in practice?

You prepare the list of actions to be performed. This final list will include everything that we could have done differently than what we were used to, behave differently than what we were used to, respond differently than what we were used to or speak differently than what we were used to. This list can only be prepared after we have prepared the previous lists. There are no shortcuts. There is no option of skipping over the stages. The previous lists (internal and regarding our inner emotional and mental landscape), are those that pave the way towards the actual actions and their implementation in practice. To return for the final time to this cruel boss of ours, here are a few examples for optional behavioral changes:

*Behave differently* – Stop cursing him or wishing him an early death every time we leave his room or conclude a conversation with him. Stop gossiping and dissing him to our work colleagues in every meeting in the hall or at the coffee machine.

*Act differently* -- Show some compassion towards him. Be more empathic towards him. Raise streamlining proposals that will change the situation in the organization to the benefit of everyone, such as bonding and enjoyable team spirit-building activities outside the office. Find a way to make him feel better about himself.

*Respond differently* – No more eye rolling or dramatic sighs. Offer help instead. Be more attentive and better listeners. Bitch and whine less.

*Speak differently* – Speak to him in a pleasant and / or respectful tone or just more calmly in order to soothe him and improve his responses. Occasionally show appreciation for his investment in his employees and his contribution to the company.

As we will find ourselves doing new things which are somewhat different than what we are used to, it is recommended to do them even if some of them initially feel "fake." Do them even if they feel "unnatural." Do them even if it "isn't even our job." Do them even if some part of us screams, "But what about us? We are entitled too!" Do them even if we feel that we are not getting anything out of it. Do them because we are not engaging in this flurry of new activity because we are suckers or because we are not true to ourselves or because we are losing ourselves (which is what our ego usually tells us). The opposite is true. We are finally seeing the big picture from a bird's-eye view, seeing the entire path our life has taken and which we wish to take. We are finally looking at the long-term; we are final leaving the boundaries of our own skin. Most importantly, we are finally taking into account our supreme good and our self-growth from the perspective of reconnecting with and establishing a mutually beneficial relationship with the part within us that knows what we are really here to accomplish. When we succeed in changing how we think, how we feel and what we do, we change reality. We progress, we evolve and we are rewarded for those changes in the shape of a generally good feeling, a filling sense of satisfaction, a sensation of soothing existential security and an increased frequency in our moments of happiness and joy.

## *Summary of the third question – what can we change?*

- This practical question takes the theoretical insights gained from the answers of the first two questions and places them *into the reality of our material life,* into our everyday lives that includes our thoughts, our emotions and our actions.

- *The key word is will* – We must want to change and be changed.

- If we want to change our situation, we must *assume responsibility* for it -- both for creating it (and the understanding that we create the reality of our life for the most part without being aware of it) and for leaving it (and the specific actions leading us there).

- *Changing what we think:* We can change how we perceive our situation by:

  1. Acting out of *self-awareness and separation* from the specific situation.
  2. *Concentrating the data*: A list of benefits, a list of supreme and lower subconscious reasons that led to the formation of this situation and a list of reflections. The answers to these questions are, in and of themselves, the solutions.
  3. *Listing new perceptions* (a combination of spiritual perceptions and our supreme good).

- *Changing how we feel:* Our thoughts and emotions are interwoven, affect each other and are affected by each other. That is why we must change how we feel towards the situation by:

  1. *Identifying and confessing the emotion.*
  2. *A conscious wish* to change that emotion.
  3. *Cleaning and draining the negative emotions* out of us.
  4. *A true appreciation* of the opportunity presented to us by the situation in the form of thankfulness.

*The way to make changes is from the inside outwards. That is the proper order of things.* The inner change we performed in our thoughts and our emotions is what enables an outer change in behavior.

- *Changing our actions and behavior:* The stage where we move from words to actions, from inner changes to outer changes, with the *list of new actions.* What can we do differently? How can we behave differently? How can we react differently? How can we speak differently?

- Seeing the bigger picture from a bird's-eye perspective, looking at the long-term, leaving the boundaries of "me," referring to our supreme good, our growth and the establishment of a mutually beneficial relationship with the part within us that knows what we are here to accomplish, will lead to a change in the reality of our lives, a generally better feeling, a sense of satisfaction and existential security and more frequent moments of happiness and joy in our lives.

# Case studies
## Stories from the clinic and from life

This chapter contains ten separate illustrations of the implementation of the trilogy method on specific cases meant to provide you with another layer of understanding, implementation and internalization of this method in your daily lives. Some of the examples provided here are chronic and deeply rooted situations that required considerable time and patience in order to understand the full picture and others are more specific situations whose solutions are relatively fast. Some of the examples presented here deal with issues considered serious and essential, whereas others deal with lighter daily issues. Most of these cases were discussed in the clinic itself whereas others (cases 3 and 10) were analyzed with the trilogy method by people who were asked to assist in the writing of this chapter by sharing challenges they had to face.

**Case Study 1** – "Hates Doing Homework" – about a mother who hates helping her son prepare his homework assignments.

**Case Study 2** – "The Lump in My Uterus is Back" – about a woman who is facing a large lump in her uterus which is reappearing for the second time in her life.

**Case Study 3** – "Maturing towards a Relationship" – about a man who cannot persist in his relationships and keeps on looking for the perfect woman for himself.

**Case Study 4** – "Stuck at Home while Pregnant" – about a woman fired from her workplace at the beginning of her first pregnancy who cannot find work.

**Case Study 5** – "Bankruptcy"-- about a woman and her coping with the painful bankruptcy of her husband's business.

**Case Study 6** – "Economic Crisis" – about a man experiencing a severe economic crisis and his coping with the fears that this event raises in him.

**Case Study 7** – "My Husband is the Cook" – about a woman who hates to cook and needs to feed her daughter when she returns from school.

**Case Study 8** – "A Painful Breakup with a Business Partner" – about a man whose business partner decides, without prior warning, to end their partnership.

**Case Study 9** – "Registration for School" – about a mother who cannot register her daughter to her school of choice.

**Case Study 10** - "I'm Infected with HIV" – about a man who is infected with the HIV virus and becomes a carrier who must face rejection.

## Case Study 1 *"Hates Doing Homework"*

### Background

Michal, a mother of two sons, had a "deep hatred" as she put it, of reviewing her younger son's homework with him. This is her second son. He is in the second grade and has a very hard time maintaining his concentration for over ten minutes, a hard time understanding the taught material and a hard time writing things down. Her frustration existed on several levels: firs She did not understand why her eldest son (who was in fifth grade), did not have any problems. He was very responsible, very intelligent and everything went smoothly for him. All she had to do was check his notebooks every few days and rejoice in his accomplishments. It was really almost no work at all. Michal felt that the nightmare of helping her second child prepare his homework was a type of unjust punishment forced upon her for the future (until his matriculation from high school at age 18). This situation harmed her relationship with her second son since during their homework preparation she became impatient with him and quite frequently found herself at wits end, screaming her head off at him. Though she promised herself every day that this time she would keep control of herself and be more patient – she found herself unable to keep that promise. Her impulses and the situation simply overwhelmed her.

The mere thought of spending the afternoon helping her son prepare his homework raised unpleasant sensations and she would blame herself for the bad situation. She felt that something as wrong with her and that was why she was a bad mother. Furthermore, her frustration led to friction and irritation with her husband who worked late every night and was barely present at home during the evenings. Worse, he also kept on lecturing her saying, "This is your job, there is no choice and I really don't see why it is so difficult to spend a few minutes each day with the child on his homework." These lectures did not, of course, improve things and led to repeated confrontations between them.

1. **Finding the "silver lining:"** (What are the benefits? What do we get? What do we learn?)

"I make up for it in other ways:" -- This difficulty pushes me to be a more accepting, hugging and calm mother whenever I am not helping him with his homework. I barely shout or become angry and I maintain better self-control whenever I am not involved with the homework.

"Grades are not the most important thing:" -- I understand that not everyone is a genius, that not everyone needs to be a straight A student. I am less fanatic in my perception of the importance of schoolwork than what I see with other parents.

"A sense of proportion in life:" -- This need to cope with my difficulty with his homework assignments changes the way I perceive things and the importance I give them. A lot of nonsense I dealt with in the past is off the table now.

"Developing patience skills:" – I am much more patient than I once was and this is expressed in other places in my life, *vis a vis* my husband and various colleagues and situations at my work place. I feel that this is "small potatoes" compared to facing the homework.

2. **Identifying the "Why?:"** (What are we missing? What is stuck / obstructed? What is not being implemented? What is striving to get out? What is being reflected upon us? Who is our mirror?)

The greatest clue for the root cause for this difficulty was a sentence that Michal repeated on several occasions: "Why is second grade homework hard to do? Nobody ever gave me any help and I got along fine in spite of not being a great genius." It turned out that as a child Michal had received no assistance or help in her studies, that she was always told she could get along on her own. Even though she faced difficulties with some of the materials, she never dared ask for help in order to avoid being thought stupid. It turned out that she was furious when she saw that her younger sister did receive help from their parents and that their mother sat with her every day. But it was important for her to please her parents and to fill the role of the successful and well-behaved daughter who could handle everything -- which is why she kept silent. Her feelings of frustration, pain and anger, which were her lot throughout her childhood, rose up and surfaced every time she sat down with her son over his homework. This aspect of Michal, this angry girl who never got any help or attention, was crying out in these situations. This was expressed in her impatience and in her lack of willingness to help and in the sense of punishment that Michal felt every day anew.

3. What to change?

**Changing how we think** (new perspectives on the situation):

Homework is no longer "my greatest nightmare." It is a chance to correct past wrongs.

"It is a great privilege to be there for my son and to help him."

"I understand how important it is to support the children, back them up and provide them with a response to their needs."

**Changing how we feel:** (What is the new emotion towards the situation? Does it include appreciation and thankfulness?)

The mixed feelings were hatred of the situation, disappointment with her mother who would only assist her sister and a general sense of frustration and helplessness. Through conversations (raising the subconscious to the conscious), writing an angry letter to her mother (there was no desire to directly confront her) and support of directed imagination in the course of which she expressed and vented out as a child all the frustration she had versus her mother and even received a response from her (in the directed imagination her mother apologized for the situation and explained that she was unaware of it and of the harsh feelings of her beloved daughter whom she always perceived as being successful). Michal was able to release all of the negative emotions that were involved in the old story and the contemporary story and even be thankful for the opportunity to right the wrong she experienced and be a different type of mother.

**Changing what we do:** (How can we act differently? Behave differently? Respond differently? Speak differently?)

"As soon as I vented out all of the anger and frustration of which I was unaware, I found myself calmer and more serene. Most importantly, the desire to help my son became my primary concern. I understood the importance of my support, my encouragement and strengthening the things which he was good at. This is what I do: I sit down with him patiently, stop looking at the clock every two minutes, no longer define this time as a nightmare and see it as a daily opportunity to support him one-on-one and encourage and strengthen him throughout our time together. Furthermore, I understood that I was repeating the same errors that I had suffered from with my eldest son by assuming that he was doing fine on his own because everything was going so easily for him. I began spending more quality time with him as well, asking him if he needed help. I feel that I have become a better mother"

## Case Study 2 "The Lump in My Uterus Is Back"

### Background

Sarit, 50 years old, married for 30 years and a mother of 4. Sarit married her husband out of love and with great joy in having left the sibling-filled house in which she grew up and in which she felt neglected over so many years.

During the first ten years of her marriage, Sarit suffered from both physical and verbal violence from her husband and psychological abuse by his family (who constantly humiliated and shamed her). Her husband was a workaholic who left her to raise the children on her own. Their relationship was bad and characterized by considerable violence (daring to express an opinion contrary to his own would result in a beating) and with many affairs on his part which resulted in battering (when she found notes and hints of affairs he had and dared to confront him about it). The first sign of change occurred after one of her brothers filed a complaint about him to the police and the husband agreed to undergo treatment instead of going to prison. The physical violence ended but the verbal violence and humiliations continued. She attempted to leave several times over the years but they all ended with his promises that he would change and she came back home. Her father, with whom she had a powerful connection and who served as an anchor for her, passed away three years ago and Sarit, whose greatest source of strength was gone and who no longer had anyone to lean on, felt abandoned and alone.

The second change occurred a year later when a lump was found in her uterus. She was operated on and the lump was removed. The recuperation period was difficult as she received no support from her husband. "We lived in two separate worlds. His world simply was not connected to mine. I felt he was not mine. When I embraced him, I felt that other women had a piece of him as well but he always denied this and told me that I was delirious, possessive and jealous and that I had mental issues."

Something began to awaken in Sarit and she began a process of empowerment in whose framework she began to study energetic healing, began an emotional-psychological treatment, slowly empowered herself and began to appreciate herself. Her husband disparaged her and mocked the processes but she carried on and ignored him. The change was good for her. She began receiving positive feedback from the environment and she even began providing energetic healing to others with positive and even astounding results soon following.

After about two years of empowerment and strengthening, the lump showed up again, in the same place as before, accompanied by the same pains. It could be felt by touch, since it was the size of a tennis ball. An operation was scheduled a month after the discovery. This time, in spite of the fears and the worries that came up, including the painful fact that her husband still did not support her in the process, Sarit decided to dig in and discover the root cause for the lump's reappearance in the womb, of all places. Furthermore, she began to focus on herself and to undergo a complete energetic-spiritual treatment of all of the relationships in her life.

1.  **Identifying the "silver lining:"** (What are the benefits? What do we get? What do we learn?)

"This a wakeup call! I am important" -- I understand that if I do not stand up and look after myself, no one else will. A string belief is growing in me that I can beat this.

"I focused in on myself in order to find myself" – I understand how important my work on myself, caring for myself, feeling important to myself, empowering myself is, regardless of what the people around me think.

"I was able to create a separation between myself and my husband" – he is not with me in this story. He is still living in his own world. For the first time, I am able to tell myself, "Let him do whatever he wants, I exist on my own account and not through him."

"I stopped complaining and whining to the entire world" – For years I shared with those around me with how badly off I was. This time I am leaving it to myself. I do not want to negativity. I do not want the negativity to gain more energy.

"I was able to wean myself off of over-reporting" – I have no more need to advertise every little detail. It does not really contribute anything, does not really alleviate anything and does not really help. It is nothing more than prattling that takes me out of myself.

"I don't involve my children with my pain as much as I used to" – Anxiety has always led me to over-share with them how badly I felt and to overburden them. This time I felt that there was no need to share my fears and anxieties about the operation with them.

2. **Identifying the "Why?:"** (What are we missing? What is stuck / obstructed? What is not being implemented? What is striving to get out? What is being reflected upon us? Who is our mirror?)

In her internal investigation as to the reasons for the appearance of the lump in the uterus of all places, Sarit found three different and complementary insights. The first – "uterus = tomorrow." (In Hebrew the two words are an anagram). From a place of daily anxiety and survival throughout her life, Sarit worried about what tomorrow would bring. Would he leave her? Would he go on humiliating her? How many other women will he have? When will he share with her what he is doing with all of the money? Until when will she continue living life like this? "I understood that I had to start dealing with the here and now and let tomorrow be. I needed to cut myself off from all of these thoughts that were driving me mad and wouldn't let me be and started dealing with what was happening with me here and now." Her second insight was that uterus = femininity. Systematically and over many years, through humiliation and cheating, her husband offended her femininity and trampled it underfoot: "I no longer remembered what it was to feel like a sexy woman with passions and healthy appetites, to feel that I was a real and valuable woman. I had to go back to feeling all this anew, regardless of what he thought of me." The third insight was related to giving. Uterus = motherhood = unconditional giving: "I gave so much to the entire world (to my children, my husband, my family and my friends) and I had nothing left for myself. I did not really think I deserved anything either. From now on, I intend to carefully select and prioritize what I give -- first comes me and then everything else."

Furthermore, Sarit understood the reflections that her husband reflected at her through his infidelity, contempt and lack of faith in her: "I didn't actually believe in myself, I didn't believe in my abilities. To say that I underestimated myself would be putting it mildly. I felt that I was nothing, that I was just another household item to be manhandled regardless of its own desires, that I was nothing more than a decorative vase. I was therefore afraid to get up and leave – because who was I without him? What I saw and experienced on the outside was deep within me and it was time to begin to believe in myself again, to get to know myself again and to love what I discovered. This had nothing to do with him anymore, just with me."

After about a month of intensive work on herself and a day before her appointment at the clinic to prepare her for surgery, Sarit's husband came home one evening and asked to speak with her. Absent any early warning, over an entire hour he opened his heart to her and for the first time came clean regarding all of his infidelities. With softness and honesty, which she had never encountered in all of their thirty years together, he told her about everything he had been through and was going through and how she was the most important person in the world for him. He told her that she was the best woman in the world, that he now understood the mistakes he had made and that he sincerely apologized for them. After the initial shock, Sarit, instead of shouting and screaming at him as she had always done in the communications between them, she responded as if she was a completely different person. She calmly told him that she was glad that he came clean, that she was proud of his honesty and initiative but what was important was what would happen from now on. Her husband responded that he was done with this chapter in his life and that from now on she was the only one he wanted. Although she had already heard endless promises from him for change in the past, this time something really felt different and they went to sleep together embraced.

The next morning, Sarit went to the clinic to undergo the examinations prior to the operation scheduled two days later. *The examination, however, revealed that the lump was gone. The ultrasound also displayed no sign of it. The lump was simply gone.* The astounded doctor who examined Sarit did not know how to explain the amazing finding but Sarit knew deep in her heart what had happened and in that moment she felt that her connection to the Creator of the Universe had been restored.

3.  What to change?

**Changing how we think** (new perspectives on the situation)

"I am important" – I am in a different place in life. I have full faith in myself, in my power, in the Creator of the Universe and in my own abilities.

"I found myself and he found his own way back to me" -- as soon as I stopped directing all of my energy at my husband

and began to nurture, empower and conserve my energy, his energy was attracted back to mine.

"I am feminine and sexy" -- I got my femininity back. I am a feminine, sexy and desirable woman.

"I choose to stay with my husband out of a place of strength" -- In the past, I stayed with my husband out of weakness and out of a sense of worthlessness. It is clear to me that other women in my position would have chosen to leave him but today I am a strong woman and I choose to remain in order to help him make his own self-correction.

"My purpose is to empower other women" – I discovered my purpose in life. Suddenly girls, teenagers and women who feel like victims and who are often victimized and are in a very bad place in their lives are coming to me. I know exactly what they are going through and what they are feeling and experiencing and I treat them and empower them.

**Changing how we feel:** (What is the new emotion towards the situation? Does it include appreciation and thankfulness?) "I am happier, I feel better and I really enjoy my newfound self-confidence. I speak to the women who come to me and I know where they are coming from. Every such story reminds me of where I was and where I will never return. I had to go through it all in order to reach the amazing place where I am now and therefore not only do I not feel any anger, but I also feel thankfulness to the Creator of the World to whom I feel fully connected now, who directed things in the best possible way for me and helped me find myself. To return to myself. To feel whole about myself again."

**Changing what we do:** (How can we act differently? Behave differently? Respond differently? Speak differently?)
"I allow others to help me" – Suddenly my husband is helping around the house, is cleaning a little, is helping with shopping, is investing more of himself in the household and I allow all this to happen.

"I am no longer cursing and screaming" – I have vented out all of my inner frustrations and I therefore no longer feel the need to lash out at anyone. I am much calmer.

"Communication between us has changed" – I no longer reply to my husband in an unpleasant way as I did in the past. My tone of voice has changed and became calmer. For example, if in the past he would complain about my cooking, because I was so filled with rage, a single word from him was enough to unleash a World War. Today I am calm and I just ignore such remarks. In general, we talk more openly about things.

"I don't have to agree to sex" – In the past, I agreed every time my husband wanted sex. I collected every crumb he gave me just so I would feel he was giving me something from himself. Today, if I do not feel like it then I listen to myself and tell him, "No." Since I accept myself, he accepts how I am with understanding.

"I built myself an energy-based treatment room" – I finally have my own corner in the house. As soon as I found a place within me that appreciates and treasures my abilities, it has shown up on the outside as well.

"I began to eat healthy and to pay attention to what I put inside of my body" – I take care of myself and suddenly this is not a nightmare or hard work. I am losing weight without suffering and I look much healthier.

"The cleanliness and orderliness of the house no linger occupies my mind all day" – I finally let it go. I have other and more important things to deal with.

"I thank the Creator of the World through celebrating the Shabbat." – I am not religious in any way but preparing the home for the Shabbat is my personal way of thanking the creator for what he has done for me. (

"There is greater harmony in the household." – The communications between the family members has changed since my inner harmony reflects on everyone.

## *Case Study 3 "Maturing Towards a Relationship"*

### Background

Daniel is a 36-year-old spiritual mentor who has been helping people discover and realize their purpose. However, Daniel himself has yet to find the special someone in his life. It has been two years since he was in any long-term romantic relationship and he defines this period as maturation preparatory for the relationship that is right for him.

In his childhood and his teenage years, the whole subject of relationships frustrated him since he was both chubby and shy and since he had many good-looking and seemingly romantically successful friends which did not contribute to his self-esteem or self-confidence: "I thought that I was incomplete without a relationship with a woman and that perhaps something was wrong with me." At the age of 18, once involved with his first girlfriend, his frustration began to loosen up since "finally someone had chosen me, wanted me. I was worth something." With time and experience and to no small extent thanks to the fact that he was employed as a barman, Daniel's self-image continued to strengthen and he experienced quite a few romantic and sexual relationships.

At the age of 25, he found himself with a great love that lasted three years until the painful moment when his heart broke when he found out that she was cheating on him: "I really felt like my heart was crushed and this impacted the relationships in my life for a long time." Since then, he has had around ten short-term relationships, none of them lasting more than six months, in which a repetitive pattern occurred.

He got the women to break up with him (by distancing himself) because "I don't have the balls to break up with them." What underlies this pattern is his fear of being hurt again: "I don't open up completely in order to avoid getting hurt because when I give of myself, I get hurt."

1. **Identifying the "silver lining:"** (What are the benefits? What do we get? What do we learn?)

"First of all, I accept myself." -- That is the greatest benefit. The understanding that I do not need anything external to be happy. That is a real experience for me and not a mere thought. Today I know that everything is all right with me.

"I am ripening" – There is a law of nature regarding "ripeness." If an orange takes six months to ripen, then I, as a human being, take 36 years to ripen. There is incredible precision here which always works in my supreme best interest.

"An unripe fruit will pair up with an unripe fruit." – A relationship, in my eyes, should be between two people who are growing spiritually and who are always in harmony. In the past, I was with women who were unripe spiritually which created a dependence that did not work. Both of us, my intended one and I, are maturing in parallel.

"When I know perfection, she will appear." -- Because I will not find anything in her that does not exist in me. That is a very significant lesson in life which provides a great deal of peace and quiet.

2. **Identifying the "Why?:"** (What are we missing? What is stuck / obstructed? What is not being implemented? What is striving to get out? What is being reflected upon us? Who is our mirror?)

Over the past five years, Daniel has been working on opening the chakra of the heart. "It is like peeling an onion; you can't accelerate the process because it has its own pace." Only now does he feel ready to undergo the final release of past hurts. Daniel's past hurts stem from two traumatic periods: His first love at the age of 18 and the infidelity of his girlfriend at the age of 25. At the age of 18, after his first girlfriend, Daniel fell into a depression. During the relationship, he found himself in a significant state of cognitive dissonance – on the one hand, a great desire to love and be loved and on the other hand, an aversion to love. He began to feel that something was wrong but did not know how to identify it. When he began his therapy process, he also examined previous incarnations and found that he was previously injured in his heart Chakra (as a Native American chief who was slain by an arrow fired at his heart). He also found out that he had experienced additional incarnations that ended with the injury of his heart. This discovery helped him emotionally understand both the depression he felt and the deep hurt he felt at the infidelity he experienced at the age of 25. "This pain is still in the system. I haven't cleaned it out enough and I am working on it now." The injured, betrayed and angry aspect in Daniel's soul, that aspect which refuses to enter into a relationship again and which led Daniel to avoid his partners as soon as their relationship reached a certain stage, has yet to receive the attention it requires for the years that have passed. It now seeks it in the way he expresses himself and in the way he vents out his anger and fears. Furthermore, Daniel realizes that in the depths of his spirit and soul exists a belief that a romantic relationship = betrayal, that opening his heart = vulnerability. These beliefs played a significant role in obstructing romantic relationships in his life and he is treating them in order to let them go and express new beliefs on relationships and an open heart. "I now understand the dissonance between the incredible power of the heart and how it closes up – *It is so powerful on the one hand and so vulnerable on the other*. And yet, when the heart is open, you act differently and behave differently and this is associated not only with relationships but in all fields of life. So it is important for me to be with someone who, like me, already treated herself and is no longer lugging around old injuries or betrayal-induced scars."

3. What to change?

**Changing how we think:** (new perspectives on the situation)

"Everything is precisely calibrated for my good, even right now." – I just need to enable it to be.

"Everything already exists right here. Here, here, here!!!" -- Unlike the "Where is she???" I think and I say: "Here she is.

She's right here."

"The color I smear on the white canvas will become the complete painting." – We are all a frequency. A vibration. That is what we really are. And when I live the vibration required for a relationship, I become a relationship.

"If it's not a big yes, it's a big no." – When it happens it will be nothing less than overwhelming and that is the place I release my doubts and questions.

**Changing how we feel:** (What is the new emotion towards the situation? Does it include appreciation and thankfulness?)

In addition to cleansing and draining the negative feelings that remained in his system from the hurtful infidelity, Daniel works daily on the connection between his emotions, thoughts and frequencies that he broadcasts out into the world: "Emotion is, at the end of the day, a byproduct of thought. So if I think, "Here she is!" That automatically makes me feel stability, harmony, joy, pride, connectivity, knowledge, security and love. When I am focused on the desired emotions – I become that emotion. When that happens, the frequency and then the law of gravity provide me with evidence that everything is well, and how close it is like the reflections I see in the women I have been dating lately. It is coming really close to what I want and it is becoming more and more precise."

**Changing what we do:** (How can we act differently? Behave differently? Respond differently? Speak differently?)

I choose to perform the following actions that strengthen the desired thoughts:

I buy my love gifts.
I check out vacation homes for two online.
I buy her tiny slippers and put them in my room.
I bought a pleasant feminine perfume and I daubed some around the room so that I would be exposed to the scent of a woman.
I "work" on my subconscious so that my "couple" frequency will grow increasingly stronger.

## Case Study 4 "Stuck at Home while Pregnant"

### Background

Osnat, 30-years-old, is the mother of a tiny baby. Osnat arrived at the clinic for her therapy with her child. She was extremely irritated after a year-long period of "being stuck at home without work." She became pregnant about ten days after her wedding: "I always yearned for this moment and I was sure that it would flood me with positive feelings because I finally created life with my beloved." However, about two months after the desired pregnancy began, the company she worked for went bankrupt and Osnat found herself at home. This event was highly traumatic for her since she had worked ever since she could remember and "never knew what rest was." She always trusted herself and only herself. In a single moment she lost her financial independence and had to bid her ability to provide for herself farewell. During her pregnancy she was forced to withdraw savings that she had accumulated throughout her life in order to survive the tough period. She had thoughts such as: "How can I not work? What will I do with this spare time? How can we survive financially with only one salary?" These troubled her day and night. She was not comforted by thinking that the man she married would provide for their family or that she was pregnant with a child she had yearned for: "It was supposed to fill me up but I felt that my entire world had been upended." Osnat was filled with anger during her pregnancy, after the birth and during her maternity leave. Her joy with the entry of her son into her life and becoming a mother was tinged with considerable anger towards herself and the entire world. Thoughts such as: "How is this happening to me? Why is this happening to me? I am a good person." clouded her thought this entire period. When Osnat reached the clinic, she had already been trying for a good long while to get back on the job market and find work in the field of marketing in which she was trained -- even though she did not really enjoy it or want to be active in it. She had completed a master's degree in organization development but it was hard to enter this field without prior experience which was why she never attempted to seek a position in this field.

1.  **Identifying the "silver lining:"** (What are the benefits? What do we get? What do we learn?)

"My man really is taking care of me." -- Since the death of

her father at a young age, a death that was very traumatic for her, Osnat never really trusted anyone else in regards to finances or anything else. This period was an opportunity to prove to herself that she really could rely on someone else, an opportunity that would not have arisen in any other way.

"I can loosen up a bit and not take responsibility for everything." – Not everything had to be on her shoulders. The excessive responsibility she assumed never gave her a chance to stop and rest.

"It turns out that the world does not collapse if I do not work." -- Osnat believed that the day she would no longer be able to work would be the end of the world. This fear motivated her for years. Now, facing her greatest fear, she realized that the world still stood.

"I can focus on what I really want to do." – As long as she was looking for a job, why not take advantage of the opportunity to try to enter the field she had always desired?

2. **Identifying the "Why?"** (What are we missing? What is stuck / obstructed? What is not being implemented? What is striving to get out? What is being reflected upon us? Who is our mirror?)

"The universe was signaling to me that I was grounded because I needed a moment to stop and reflect and recalculate my course -- a moment of reflection my hectic schedule never had room for." Since her father's death, Osnat never gave herself a moment to think, to process events which had occurred to her throughout her life, to understand what she really wanted to do with her life, to find out what her true desires were and who she really was. "The path I specialized in over the years was the 'path of escape' and something within cried out, "No more!" Osnat finally dared to touch upon the traumatic wound left by the death of her father and release the enormous pain of abandonment interwoven into it. Another issue that floated to the surface during her therapy was letting go. Osnat was a "control freak." This was expressed by the need to control every detail of her life and her obsession with orderliness and cleanliness. She was able to see how her absence of control in everything having to do with her father's death led her, out of an instinct of self-preservation, to assume the other extreme of control.

Another aspect had to do with her purpose in life: "I always knew, deep inside, that my purpose was to help people and help businesses do better." Life's circumstances led her down a detour that prevented her from reaching the self-fulfillment for which she yearned. Her current obstruction rekindled the fire in her heart and she dared to once again dream about making a living by helping people and their businesses.

3. **What to change?**

**Changing how we think:** (new perspectives on the situation) "Only thanks to my time off can I reconnect to myself." – This is not the greatest disaster that ever happened to me.

"This is the right time for me to stop, digest and let go." -- I had to go through this. Of course I did not think so for a very long time but everything that happened, happened for my supreme good.

"I deserve to enjoy life a little." – Life is not just having a job and making a living. I can begin to enjoy my family and myself.

"It is fun to be taken care of." – I enable my husband to take care of me and this is a new and pleasant sense of security that I never knew. This empowers him as well.

**Changing how we feel:** (What is the new emotion towards the situation? Does it include appreciation and thankfulness?) Osnat was angry at her situation, at herself and the mother she unwillingly became for a long, long time: "I had a new child and for a very long time what he got was an angry mother who was disappointed with herself, who wasn't fully committed with all her heart to motherhood." Identifying the sources of the anger and fear which motivated Osnat for so many years and consciously expressing them released her emotional waste and let in compassion for herself. The situation enabled her to learn how to love herself again without defining herself by her career and this enabled her to fall in love with her son with all of her heart.

**Changing what we do:** (How can we act differently? Behave differently? Respond differently? Speak differently?)

Osnat began to feel more and more comfortable at home (no longer feeling like a miserable victim stuck at home) and became patient, calm and more loving with her husband and son. She even began to send out resumes to a number of open positions, not only in the field of marketing, but also in the field of organizational consultancy. These efforts soon bore fruit -- only a few months into the process. In response to one of her resumes, the opportunity of working for a huge company in a challenging position that included managing mid-level managers and junior workers, within a department that was undergoing a process of organizational consulting, arose. It was not a proper organizational consulting position, but the possibility of being part of this process in a large and well-known company intrigued and thrilled her. This was exactly the field experience she was missing and wished to sample. Osnat returned to the labor market different, more complete, more connected, calmer, more liberated and most importantly more accepting of reality and the challenges it held: "I can always choose to remember what had happened, what I went through and how it affected me. I decide not to go back to that dark place. The time I spent at home, in spite of the difficulties it involved, allowed me to look within myself and find Osnat again. To love myself as I am."

## Case Study 5 "Bankruptcy"

### Background

Sigal, was a 40-year-old mother of two children, a son and a daughter, happily married for many years to her much beloved husband. Her husband had a business in the food sector and she was a salaried employee in a private company. One day, like thunder on a clear day, her husband informed her that the business had to file for bankruptcy. He had invested many years, many hours (mostly at the expense of the family) and much money (All of their savings and various loans in this business) running his business. Suddenly, creditors were banging at their doors. Their car and bank accounts were foreclosed; their credit cards were frozen; her husband was mortified with shame and she herself was overwhelmed with existential fear.

1. **Identifying the "silver lining:"** (What are the benefits? What do we get? What do we learn?)

"An understanding that we weren't really open with one another." -- He never really told me what was going on with the business and I did not ask in order not to know. It was convenient for me to ignore the signs. This situation forced us to sit down and talk, to be open with one another, to share.

"I understood what was truly important in life -- love, a roof over our head and food on our plate." – Sigal had a long-standing aversion to the house that she had lived in her entire life -- one which she had inherited. She hated it and constantly dreamed of the day that they would leave it. Following the crisis, the house quickly became the only safe anchor, the only stable ground. Suddenly she began to appreciate it and ceased to take it for granted. She found she had love and the ability to put food on the table and that sufficed.

"The children got their father back and I got support." – Suddenly Dad was at home. After years of dedicating himself to the business and barely being at home, suddenly he was there, preparing food for his children, sitting down with his child to prepare homework, being involved in their ongoing life and, in particular, as an active partner in the maintenance of the household.

"I got help from people I never imagined would be there for me and from people whom I never counted as close to me." There was the former boss who gave me a car until I was able to get back on my feet again and my mother suddenly became the figure I most trusted in the world after years of a charged and not simple relationship.

"The situation provided me with a stage to display the love of those around me." -- There was a lot of positive feedback from the environment about how I was courageously dealing with the situation.

"I am here too and I deserve things as well." -- I understand that I am a person before I am a mother and a wife. I find that I allow myself to do things that are only for me, in spite of, and, even because of, the difficult situation. For example, I don't return home right after work and I go out with friends or I just wander around the mall in order to window shop.

"I began to produce and sell jewelry." – The situation encouraged me to develop an additional income channel. Over time, the excellent feedback and the sales, I found out that I like this activity as a hobby but not as a job in and of itself. That, too, was an important insight.

2.  **Identifying the "Why?"** (What are we missing? What is stuck / obstructed? What is not being implemented? What is striving to get out? What is being reflected upon us? Who is our mirror?)

"The reason for the creation of the situation was a kind of a slap in the face that I received in order to wake me up and give me the opportunity to change my life. I was not even aware that my life needed a change." Sigal did not think that she was lacking anything. After all, she had a mortgage-free home (even though she hated it), she had wonderful children and she had a husband she truly loved. However, in practice she lacked many things: She lacked recognition and appreciation for everything she had – her daily routine was filled with complaints about driving the children to their after-school activities, about her mother and the job she hated. Her relationship lacked openness and sharing and the ability to discuss things as they were, in spite of the great love between her and her husband. (This understanding shocked her and even momentarily cracked her faith in her spouse.) There was a lack of recognition and thankfulness for having her own house. She was so busy hating it and hating the fact that she was "stuck in it," that only the trepidation that she felt at the thought of losing it could shake her out of that hatred. She missed having a calm and serene husband – stressful calls from the bank, returning home late, intense stress and troubled sleep from worries were his daily routine over the past years and this was expressed at her expense and the expense of the children.

"I lacked the courage, strength, self-love, self-fulfillment and an understanding of essence rather than matter. I only received all these thanks to facing the situation." Sigal never really loved herself. She truly wanted to but she seemingly never found anything to love about herself, anything particularly worthwhile or special about her, which is why she always put herself last in the family's priorities. Everyone's needs were more important than her own.

3. **What to change?**

**Changing how we think:** (new perspectives on the situation) "Appearances don't really matter." – The jeep was foreclosed and exchanged for an older vehicle. I understood that the only thing that mattered was having a vehicle with an air conditioner that ran.

"Together we can get through anything." – I repeat this mantra every day. We are not the only people this happened to and the main thing was being able to face these things together, not only with my husband but also with my mother.

"I am strong and I can do anything." – Every time a call comes from a lawyer or more negative news regarding the bankruptcy, I permit myself to be sad for a few minutes and then I find my focus and recall my strength.

"I never lose, I either win or I learn." – That is a sentence I repeat to myself as part of my general approach towards adopting a positive way of thinking. I choose to focus on what is good and what is present.

"I have great reserves of power." – I managed to use this opportunity to learn, grow and understand not to adopt a victim mentality. This indicates power, a quality I never would have attributed to myself.

"It is all under control." – Knowing this deep in my heart is the most empowering feeling there is.

**Changing how we feel:** (what is the new emotion towards the situation? Does it include appreciation and thankfulness?)
Sigal felt a great deal of anger at her husband about "How could he do this to us?"and at herself for never asking, "What is really going on with the business?" and for looking the other way (in spite of her hunches) and at the situation itself. "Why do my children need to be hurt like this?" She understood,

however, that if she hurled all of her anger at her husband, this would not be productive. Accordingly, she decided to express and vent her anger in creative and non-harmful ways such as talking during therapy, writing, guided imagination and developing compassion towards her husband. She placed herself in his shoes, empathizing with his disappointment with himself, his feeling of failure and his pain at the shattering of his dreams. She shared her own feelings with him in carefully selected moments and the proper ambience and found that her words were heard and penetrated better -- without unnecessary conflict.

**Changing what we do:** (How can we act differently? Behave differently? Respond differently? Speak differently?)
"I no longer permit my fear of knowing to paralyze me." – I refuse to be scared at receiving answers because I know we will get through whatever we need to get through together.

"I thought about a million creative ways to maintain a stable home." – At first, the thought of not having a credit card or money to shop or to pay for extra-curricular classes for the children and of the other basics kept me sleepless at night. But I made sure that my children would never feel that anything in our lives had changed.

"Today we talk about everything." – A new level of communication has emerged between us. I both express myself and ask for and receive answers. I refuse to give that up.

"I transformed my house into my home with all my heart." – In the past, I did not even want to take care of it since I hated it and I never invited people home to my place. Given the situation, I showered it with loving care: I painted it, I put up curtains and I made all sorts of tiny but significant touches. It is suddenly fun to be in the house and it is suddenly fun to be visited in the house.

"I permit myself to cry." – I tell myself that I am allowed to let go but I am not swallowed up by it and I refuse to slide down into victimhood because I keep on reminding myself of the three most important things that I do have: Love (of all kinds), a roof to sleep under and food to put on our plates.

"I brought honesty and loyalty to myself into my life." – I am not afraid to say what I think. Instead of eating my heart and my head out, I express myself and share. I do this in all fields of life -- at work, with friends, families and my husband.

## Case Study 6 "An Economic Crisis"

### Background

Shay, a 50-year-old man, happily married and father of three, owned a private business that provided consultation and strategy formation services which yielded a respectable income. The business provided a high standard of living for himself and his family. However, suddenly and without warning, Shay found himself in the midst of a severe financial crisis which resulted in the loss of half of his income and the profits he was used to bringing in over the years. Shay was the primary provider in his household. His wife held a part-time job, returning home in the afternoon to be with the children when they returned from their schools and kindergartens (a joint decision of both of them). Accordingly, he felt his world had collapsed. He did not know how he would meet all of the many expenses and regular payments they had. This difficult situation lasted over five months out of which, for about two months: "I was stuck in a kind of frightening paralysis. I only did what I had to do and the rest of the time, I was like a zombie. Fortunately, I benefited from therapy at the time." Shay was a skeptical and realistic person who only believed what he saw with his own eyes, and had absolutely no faith in spiritualism the occult.

1. **Identifying the "silver lining:"** (What are the benefits? What do we get? What do we learn?)

"Finding the good within the evil and focusing on it was one of the decisive factors which helped me to get out of the situation." – Every time I felt that the fear and despair were overtaking me, I remembered the impressive list I made and was able to pull myself out of these harsh sensations.

"I found out that I had no appreciation for the value and worth of money and I changed that." – For the first time in my life I understood how much I was spending without thinking and how busy I was on what I would spend my money on now and where I would spend it. I saw that I had no appreciation of the value of material possessions only after I began accounting for every penny that left my pocket.

"I allowed myself to be an informed consumer." – In the spare time I had, I did the household shopping and began to compare prices, something I had never done beforehand because I found it truly shameful.

"I spend more time with my family." – I have begun spending considerably more time with my children who accepted this rather joyfully. I am much more involved in their everyday life and I am more caring.

"I enjoy eating at home." – I found out that you do not need to subsist on gourmet meals (I had most of my business meals in restaurants in which I became a permanent resident). Cooked meals at home is something you can enjoy. This is rather new to me.

"I began to appreciate how much I really have." – I was always wrapped up with what I didn't have, what else I could buy and what I was missing. Now I suddenly discovered all of the many things I already had: A loving and healthy family, a supportive woman who has faith in me, a large house, an affluent lifestyle and considerable knowledge, experience and capabilities.

"I dared to open my mind to potential new fields of occupation." – In the past, I did not dare deviate right or left of the fields in which I was engaged. I was fixated on what I was doing. The newly available spare time I had was used to expand my horizons and for meetings and initiatives in new and unfamiliar fields.

"I suddenly won quality time to spend with my wife in the middle of the day." – Suddenly, after many years in which we had not done it, we found ourselves going to the beach together, to a daytime movie, talking and even making love in midday when there is more energy. She was very supportive of me and this reminded me of how capable I was and how much faith she had in me. This really strengthened our relationship.

2. **Identifying the "Why?"** (What are we missing? What is stuck / obstructed? What is not being implemented? What is striving to get out? What is being reflected upon us? Who is our mirror?)

Shay grew up in an affluent environment and household and was given whatever he wanted. But he was always surrounded by friends who had much more than his own family did. When he was a 20-year-old soldier, his father, who had left home three years earlier and moved in to live with a different woman, passed away from lung disease, leaving the family with heavy financial debts. For many years, Shay assumed responsibility for his mother (who was a homemaker) and his little brother and worked hard to pay back all the debts. This traumatic event shook Shay's inner world and left in him scars in the shape of anger at his father, existential anxiety and material shortages. He felt that his father had abandoned him once again and left him to "take care of all of his shit." His existential security was shaken and led to existential anxiety. This anxiety served as the motivating force that pushed him to achieve and to succeed, but also accompanied him daily and burdened him -- the fear that he would not have any money, the fear that this difficult situation would repeat itself and the fear that his family would suffer as he did. Furthermore, the desire to compensate for all of these years of want and hardship (a relative want in comparison to his childhood environment and true poverty after the death of his father), grew to high levels of wasteful expenditure and arrogance that sometimes spun out of control. "I think I created the situation or made it happen because I needed a change on several levels and had no other way to get myself to change. I changed the perception of material things in my life, false beliefs and many unhealthy habits." The difficult economic situation was, in fact, a materialization of his greatest fear and he was able to see that the end of the world did not come when it materialized. Not only was he able to overcome the situation, it made him stronger and restored his heartfelt faith in regards to everything related to his abilities.

Shay succeeded in identifying a "mechanism of paralysis." – even though it took him two months this time. But he realized that whenever change came, be it large or small, for several days his world would be painted in black, a feeling that the end of the world had arrived. It would encompass him (as it did in the past) and he would fall silent. The joyful discovery, as far as he was concerned, was that this mood was temporary and passed. Now that he was aware of his automatic response mechanism to change, he knew what he needed and wanted to change: "I discovered that paralysis and anxiety do not snap you out of the situation. On the contrary, awakening is what enables you to move, to progress and get out of it." Furthermore, Shay discovered that although he always perceived and defined himself as an optimist with great joy in life, he was in fact a pessimistic and an anxiety-filled man. Understanding the sources of this pessimistic perception and these anxieties helped him accept with compassion this unpleasant self- discovery and from there a desire to turn the scales.

3.  **What to change?**

**Changing how we think:** (new perspectives on the situation)

"My thinking needs to be optimistic rather than pessimistic." – This pessimism only causes me to sink deeper and does not help me progress.

"Whatever fate sends my way I can overcome it." – I have impressive personal capabilities that have repeatedly proven themselves throughout my life.

"This situation leads me to believe in myself, to grow and to develop."

"In the next crisis, change will come sooner." -- I know my mechanism thanks to this powerful experience and am learning how to change it.

"I am really good at what I do." – I finally believe this in my heart and not just in my head.

**Changing how we feel** (what is the new emotion towards the situation? Does it include appreciation and thankfulness?)

Shay first identified within himself an emotional storm of feeling like failure, a lack of ability and injury to his ego and self-image. For the first time, he dared express them out loud, recognize them and understand that the fact he felt this way at this moment did not really mean that this was who he was. "I understand that this is all in my own hands. I can and I should permit these emotions to rise up and I should be aware of them -- but not for more than a few days." Later on, the emotions of anger and disappointment at his father emerged as well. Since he had passed away so many years ago, Shay felt that there was no point in bringing it up or raising the pain and anger involved in it. The relief which arose following the expression of these painful feelings and their drainage, followed by his forgiving his father for not handling his business wisely and not being the business genius that Shay thought he was, proved that things were different and he had succeeded in putting this painful chapter behind him and even became grateful for the contribution of those experiences (both past and present), to his capabilities and achievements.

**Changing what we do:** (How can we act differently? Behave differently? Respond differently? Speak differently?)

"I let things be and didn't fight the situation." – I stopped being angry at the situation and wanting it to all to go away.

"It is all right to take a nap every now and again." – I let myself stay in bed and rest on those days that I was unable to get up, rather than berating myself for something being wrong with me. I found myself going to the beach in the middle of the day just for fun.
"I place limits and boundaries on my children." – I understand that I do not need to give them everything, that it is not even healthy for them for me to give them everything. I want them to learn to appreciate what they have.

"Proportionality" – a new quality that I am adopting. I no longer spend all day on the computer obsessively searching for the next vacation or placing reservations for all the newly opened restaurants.

"I compare prices." – Informed consumerism is no longer a foul word to me.

"I am taking responsibility for the situation." – I am going out, I am in motion. My next goal is to change the situation -- whether it takes a day, a week or a month.

## Case Study 7 "My Husband is the Cook"

### Background

Neta, a 35-year-old, mother of two daughters and a son, never cooks, leaving this territory to her husband. She never learned how to cook and never wanted to learn how, even though she came from an Iraqi-Jewish family where there were always "pots on the fire" and that she had a mother who was renowned for her delicious cooking. So it always was. Even when she was a young bachelorette, her family was sure that things would change when she would have her own children. Neta refused to learn to cook when additional mouths to feed were added to the household. It is not that she did nothing, no! She threw pasta into boiling water ("Fortunately, there are a million shapes and sizes which allowed me to maintain the appearance of variety.") and served it with ketchup. Sometimes she dumped one cup of rice and two cups of water with a little salt into a pan, boiled the water and scraped something resembling rice out of it. She also warmed up many animal shaped frozen schnitzels, prepared omelets and sliced up cucumbers and tomatoes to make a salad, which is how her children, whom she loved very much, got a rather basic diet of which they were actually very fond. Her husband, on the other hand, loved to cook and every evening, upon his return from work, he would prepare, for himself and for her a tasty daily hot dish. The children, however, usually refused to even taste his cooking. The fact that the kids barely ate the hot lunches prepared for them in their schools was additional proof, as far as Neta was concerned, that there was no point in making an effort because the children did not even like the "complicated foods swimming in the gravy." Together with the casseroles her mother shoved into her arms at the beginning of every week and the occasional night of Pizza-Hut or MacDonald's, Neta got along for many years without learning how to cook. This seemingly idyllic situation was overshadowed by the fact that her cooking-obsessed mother and mother-in-law refused to accept this situation, nagged her about it incessantly (each in her own way) and this resulted in quite a few arguments between them. The situation changed when two things happened simultaneously. The first change was that after many years as a salaried employee, Neta became independently employed and began working from home. At the same time, Neta's eldest daughter entered 4th grade and was no longer served a hot lunch at school. This meant she had to get a hot lunch every day when she returned from school. Just thinking about that stressed Neta. She was extremely frustrated with the new situation. The fact that she had to stand every day in the kitchen and prepare food for her daughter induced a type of stress that was expressed in actual physical tremors. When her husband tried to cheer her up by laughingly telling her: "What's the problem? One day of boot camp at your mother's and the problem is solved." She discovered that she was strongly against doing so.

1. **Identifying the "silver lining:"** (What are the benefits? What do we get? What do we learn?)

Quality time with my daughter." – We do not really sit with

each other one-on-one anymore because there are two small-er children and a lot of ruckus at home in the afternoon. It could be nice to sit down quietly and chat with her like two grownups.

"It is possible to cook and also manage a successful career." – I can prove to myself that I can be both a successful career woman and also look after my children -- that nothing comes at the expense of anything else.

"I can pamper and gladden my husband occasionally" -- even though he never said anything about it and enjoys cooking for his family, I am sure that he would be happy to come home and find a warm dish waiting for him, just like most men do.

2. **Identifying the "Why?"** (What are we missing? What is stuck / obstructed? What is not being implemented? What is striving to get out? What is being reflected upon us? Who is our mirror?)

When Neta delved deeper into the subject of cooking in her life and, more accurately, the basis of her fierce and consistent opposition to "preparing pots," two essential issues came up. The first was, "I'll do anything not to be like my mother." Her image of herself cooking up meatloaf for her daughter at noon and diving into a "What do I feel and think at that moment" caused her to admit that not only did she not really appreciate her mother throughout her life, she even despised her. She defined her as a "housewife who never did anything with her life. Her head was filled with nothing but cooking and cleaning." She felt a combination of distaste at her mother's defeatism, as she perceived it, and guilt that this is what she thought of her mother who dedicated her life to her family.

The second issue was related to her pent up rage as a girl: "All she ever gave me were pots and plates of food. What I wanted was a hug. I wanted her to pay some attention to me." From her perspective as a girl, she missed her mother's touch, the type of physical love which her mother did not know how to give. Furthermore, her mother never sat down to talk with her, to ask her how she was doing, how she was feeling. All that Neta remembered from her childhood with her mother was: "Sit down and eat honey. Who do you think I spent all these hours cooking for?" Neta needed to allow the child within her to express and release all of her anger at "these annoying pots" which never really filled in the absence of touch and attention from her mother.

3. **What to change?**

**Changing how we think:** (new perspectives on the situation)

"This is a chance for me to spend time with my daughter." – I know how much I missed it as a girl and I can give her that gift.

"A successful career need not come at the expense of my family." – I choose to combine the two.

"When I bake that meatloaf, I am baking it with love." – I also choose to express my love but not only through the stomach.

"With one action I get to make my husband, my mother and my mother-in-law happy."

**Changing how we feel:** (What is the new emotion towards the situation? Does it include appreciation and thankfulness?)

The moment Neta touched upon the sources of that resistance, she both understood them rationally and provided them with an emotional response. The anger and emotions of guilt that mostly resided on a subconscious level floated up to the conscious level, were expressed and thereby released. This gave her a great sense of relief. She needed to forgive her mother for not knowing to give her anything else aside from food. Knowing that this was simply what was common and customary at the time, that becoming a housewife was also the norm and that there was no awareness of any other possibilities in her mother's generation, helped Neta a great deal. She even understood that her desire "not to be a housewife" served as a motivating power for all of her many professional achievements. Now she was finally prepared to stop hating the pots and anything related to "mother's cooking."

**Changing what we do:** (How can we act differently? Behave differently? Respond differently? Speak differently?)
"I really fulfilled my mother's dream when I began to ask her for recipes and to show me how to cook." – It isn't that I intend

to cook complicated things, both because I have no patience for it and because I don't enjoy cooking as much as I see that my husband enjoys it. But, at least I no longer suffer and hate cooking.

"I remind myself every day how important it is and that it is not the thing that defines me and that makes me feel better."

"I hung on the refrigerator a list of simple and delicious recipes that I already know how to do." – Occasionally I add something new to the list. This does not come naturally to me and I do not have the spontaneity or the improvisation abilities natural cooks do but I am open to it and go with the flow.

"I feel closer to my mother." – An additional layer has been added to our conversations and I am gently encouraging her to expand her horizons, experience new experiences and allow herself to pamper herself more.

## Case Study 8 "A Painful Breakup with a Business Partner"

**Background**

Ziv, a 42-year-old bachelor, has managed, over the past eight years, a business partnership with Yaron in the field of entertainment project management. This partnership was based on the use of a common database and collaboration in the management and supervision of the various projects. The partnership between them moved from their business to their personal lives and they became friends. But this was never an equal partnership:

1.  It was mostly based on "Who is getting the incoming call?" It was his partner who received most of the incoming calls. Only when he was ill or over-pressured did Yaron transfer projects to Ziv.

2.  Yaron, who had a pleasant and laid-back personality, knew how to play the game and flatter their clients which made him very popular with them. Ziv, on the other hand, found it hard to be nice to people who were not nice to him and always preferred to have his high quality work speak for itself. This often led to clashes between the partners over this issue and to a number of clients who wished to work exclusively with Yaron and not with Ziv.

3.  Yaron was a dedicated businessperson who put work at the top of his priorities. Ziv, on the other hand, did not believe that one should enslave oneself to one's work too much and simply lacked the work ethic of his partner.

One day, completely out of the blue, Yaron informed Ziv that he wished to break up their partnership and end their work together at the end of that calendar year which would occur in two months. This took place in the middle of a workday while they were walking down the street in a manner that Ziv perceived to be incredibly insulting given their friendship. The trigger for the breakup as far as Yaron was concerned was a big fight between Ziv and an old client. Ziv was rather shocked since he did not expect this and, in the following days, he found himself, doing what he detested and refused to do throughout his life – beg and try to ingratiate himself with his partner in order to prevent the breakup. However, his partner was adamant about his new course and only two months of working together were left until the partnership ended. The initial shock rapidly changed to pressure and stress from the "What will happen now? What are the economic ramifications? How will I manage on my own? He brings in most of the projects" and "Some of the clients don't like me, how will I find those who do?"

1.  **Identifying the "silver lining:"** (What are the benefits? What do we get? What do we learn?)

"The endless pressure which does not suit me will finally come to an end." – Given his character, the nature of his work and the fact that he was a workaholic, Yaron kept on pressuring me and stressing me out.

"Self-criticism will either end or change." –Ziv's expectations of me led me to constantly criticize myself for not working hard enough and not trying hard enough, for not being like Ziv.

"This situation forced me to take matters into my own hands

and to begin initiating." – I really did not do much to advance the business or myself, I just let things come to me and went along with the flow.

"This is my chance to develop a personal interaction with the clients." – Even if these clients did not necessarily approach him personally but rather approached both of us as a team. Yaron would usually take over communications because I was not present enough.

"I'll stop playing second fiddle." – It is time that I stood on my own.

"I have to learn how to be nicer." – I was not able to be nice to people I do not like in the past and now I have no choice but to change.

2. **Identifying the "Why?"** (What are we missing? What is stuck / obstructed? What is not being implemented? What is striving to get out? What is being reflected upon us? Who is our mirror?)

I remained static for a long, long time and trusted in the fact that I was professional in my field and that there were not too many players at my level in the field. This is a wake-up call to get out of my sleepy comfort-zone loop." For a long time, Ziv relied on his belief that they would always have work given their professionalism and he was content with the fees he earned. However, the situation led him to understand that carrying on with the "good enough" was a type of compromise and that this was not good for him. Furthermore, he did not like the fact that he had become the "second fiddle" in this partnership, the least desired option for the clients given his abrasive character. Even though it was easy for him to pigeonhole his partner as a workaholic and to give himself a pass on putting in the extra effort, he often even found himself clashing with Yaron over his refusal to transfer projects to him when he was earning less than he was. Ziv understood that a change was required and that his partner, through his refusal to transfer projects to him, was actually reflecting to him that he had to assume responsibility for himself and his conduct. He was telling him that he had to change his work ethic and general attitude towards the people hiring their services. "He was the external criticizing and investigative eye but these were actually things that I was supposed to see on my own. For a variety of reasons it was comfortable for me not to see them."

Furthermore, Ziv was very much offended by the way his partner chose to end their partnership: "I did not expect him to be so selfish and think only about himself or that he would do it in such a cold and standoffish manner, as if there was no long-term relationship between us and, as if I was no more than an expendable product which could be thrown into the trash." The understanding that there was a very significant reflection here for him by his partner (given who he is and who he always was), helped Ziv release his anger and convert his offended feeling into a motivating force for change.

### 3. **What to change?**

**Changing how we think:** (new perspectives on the situation) "I learned that being professional was not enough in our world." – I have to emphasize the personal aspect and give more personal attention to the people with whom I work.

"The time is now ripe to wake up and do something else." – I pretty much put myself to sleep in my career development and this is a chance for me to do things differently and examine additional channels.

"I will end things with Yaron nicely." – I have made a conscious decision not to fight with him over the breakup and in the time that is left, I am making considerable efforts to change my habit of being irritated at who he is and how he acts.

"Inserting greater mental flexibility." – I am beginning to do things that I had never done before (self-promotion, reducing prices, being extra nice) and searching for more creative ways to make a living.

**Changing how we feel:** (what is the new emotion towards the situation? Does it include appreciation and thankfulness?)

"My fear of the unknown has transformed from a paralyzing force into a motivating force that gets me to the place that that is better for me, with anticipation for the new things that will come and the challenge of seeing how I can handle what life has in store for me. I love the fact that I am always bringing creative solutions to the challenges I face. There was a moment when I was already waiting for the official end of our partnership so that the feeling of relief would come and with it the positive pressure to initiate, create and renew."

This situation helped Ziv see that his way of doing things was not necessarily the best one and that his bitterness, which was expressed in his constant criticism towards Yaron and the way he "constantly bowed down to the clients," changed to an acceptance of the rules of the game backed up by the understanding that accepting them did not really lessen who he is or his professional abilities.

Furthermore, the decision not to quarrel with Yaron until the end of their partnership helped diminish Ziv's anger with Yaron. He found himself capable of greater flexibility than in the past and the ability to show greater restraint and less irritation. He even attempted to meet the other side halfway. This led to greater calmness in the communications between them. "I saw that if I could do it with him I could do it with others as well. I am truly implementing this with the communication I have with the other people with whom I interact in my job."

**Changing what we do** (How can we act differently? Behave differently? Respond differently? Speak differently?)

"I enjoy my work more." – This change restored my enjoyment

of the profession itself which had lessened over the years and with the friction that developed between Yaron and myself. It is much nicer and more pleasant at work.

"I began to approach and to court clients." – I began doing this because I had no choice and I found out that it was not nearly as terrible as I thought.

"I am more cooperative and more serene and spontaneous." – I am working for my family and myself and not for anyone else. This is bringing out the best in me. I perform various activities without being disappointed in myself as I previously was.

"I am more positive in my overall perception." – I try to meet the production halfway and help in whatever way I can. In the past, when anyone asked me for help, my automatic response was: "Damn, I don't feel like it" and I would act accordingly. Now, I put this response aside and just try to see how I can help.

"I began helping other project managers." – The desire to help has become active and I now find myself carrying out more collaborative projects -- even with my competitors. I am also looking out for myself when I do this because the time might come that I myself will need help.

"Beggars can't be choosers." – In the past, I refused to work for less money and I was very stubborn about this. Now, when I have no choice, I am more open and less defensive and so it is easier for me to take on slightly less remunerative projects.

## Case Study 9 "School Registration"

**Background**

Oshrat, 38-years-old, married and mother of three, arrived for a one-time session following a period of several weeks in which she unsuccessfully attempted to change the elementary school placement of her daughter. There were two elementary schools in the neighborhood where they lived. Her daughter was placed in the school which was considered by her to be the inferior of the two -- especially given that her daughter's kindergarten friends were placed in the preferred school and she did not want her daughter to be without old friends in her first year at school. Throughout these weeks, Oshrat sought every possible way to change the harsh municipal decision. She repeatedly went to city hall and spoke with the different parties there, used her connections in order to try to meet the mayor to discuss the matter, filed an exemption request to enter the school, seriously considered moving in order to live in an area permitted to register for this school and even took her husband to inspect apartments for rent in that area. At that point, she ran into two types of resistance – an external resistance from her aunt who refused to sign the necessary paperwork and internal resistance since this action (in the form of preparing the future lease contract to her grandfather's address) constituted a betrayal of her own values and moral system, which she held dearly. She was not really capable of going through with it.

The meeting took place several days before the conclusion

of the registration period to the schools. Oshrat arrived at it exhausted and upset due to this clash between the desire to be accepted into the school she desired and the betrayal of her value system, her refusal to accept her failure (as she saw it) and the stress that made it difficult for her to sleep at night. Even her husband refused to hear any more of it and called her behavior "not normal."

1. **Identifying the "silver lining:"** (What are the benefits? What do we get? What do we learn?)

Oshrat prepared a list of the advantage each school had and discovered that the only real advantage her preferred school had was that her daughter's friends were there. On the other hand, the list of advantages associated with the undesirable school was long:

"I will continue to live in my own home which I love so much." "This school is closer and she will be able to walk to it."

"She will learn to know a new environment and make new friends."

"I will be able to contribute everything I can to make this school better."

2. **Identifying the "Why?"** (What are we missing? What is stuck / obstructed? What is not being implemented? What is striving to get out? What is being reflected

upon us? Who is our mirror?)

In our session, we tried to dig deeper and find out why she was finding it so hard to accept the placement. Two issues came up: Acceptance and the perception of perfection. It turned out that acceptance was a very sensitive topic for her and although she herself was a very giving person, she did not really know how to receive. She both tended to deflect anything she received and she was really uncomfortable in receiving things from others, be they material objects such as gifts or abstract ones such as compliments.

Receiving something immediately caused her to feel cramps. While searching after the sources of her "difficulty to receive," it turned up that throughout her childhood she experienced feelings of rejection: "I was never accepted as a child -- who and what I was. Someone was always trying to change me: My looks (I was very pretty and they also wanted me to be really thin), my desires (if I wanted to study something, I would be met by a "Why do you need to study that?" or they just constantly told me, "So what if that is what you want?") or my choices (There was always criticism: "Why didn't you do things this way or that way?"). The rejection she experienced was on two levels -- what she wanted and who she was. This current situation forced her to deal with something she really wanted but could not have and brought the old pain of rejection into her consciousness.

The other issue which came up had to do with perfection. The desire to be accepted into the perfect school, as she perceived it, took her over to such an extent that it nearly led her to forsake her principles. In her childhood, she frequently faced the pain of "imperfection: in the form of repeated criticism: "As a child I was constantly told: "You are a pretty girl but you need to lose ten pounds." The environment kept on implying that she would not be perfect if she failed to lose those ten pounds. That is why, as a child, she experienced tremendous emotional pain since she was not really accepted as she was (Who she was not good enough) and no one really saw who she was but only what she could be. "This situation is a chance for me to deal with a situation in which my daughter is going to a school considered not as good and to see how I am dealing with it."

3. **What to change?**

**Changing how we think:** (new perspectives on the situation)

"I understood that I didn't really want what I thought I wanted." – My behavioral pattern had simply caused me to get stuck.

"I listen to the universe and to the signs around me and choose to let go." – If I try to change a given situations in so many ways and they all lead to the same result, there must be some other, stronger, force at work here and I had better let go and enable the Universe to lead me down the path which is best for me.

"I will bring all of my capabilities to the new school." – I have enormous influence and this is my chance to test how much I can change the existing reality in this school and match it to my higher standards.

"I am not a failure." – This simply was not the best path for me.

"I recognize my supreme good." – I have been given the opportunity and privilege of influencing an entire school, not just my daughter.

**Changing how we feel:** (What is the new emotion towards the situation? Does it include appreciation and thankfulness?) "As soon as I chose to change my choice, my limiting and depressing perceptions and my unease and stress cleared away and made room for emotions and sensations of excitement, curiosity at the shape of new things to come (what could be done to improve and contribute to the new school) and mostly towards acceptance of the situation which led to internal peace which I had not experienced for a long time now.

**Changing what we do:** (How can we act differently? Behave differently? Respond differently? Speak differently?)
"I am registering my daughter to the new school." – This was carried out the very day after the meeting.

"I am volunteering for the parent's committee in the school."

I will make sure that I am at home every day when she returns from school." -- This experience and all of this conformation has led me to decide to leave my current job in order to be there for her.

"I want to treat and provide a resolution for these painful childhood experiences." – Now I know where to begin and what to focus upon.

## Case Study 10 "I Was Infected With the HIV Virus"

### Background

Alon, a gay 35-year-old bachelor who loved life and lived it to the fullest found out in a routine examination that he was infected with HIV. A little over three months prior to the discovery of the infection, his father, with whom he had a difficult and complex relationship, passed away from a long illness. Furthermore, his partner for the past two years had left the country and separated from him. "I felt that my entire world had ended. I thought to myself that it was not enough that I lost the two people closest to me, I am now losing my life as well. My initial reaction was that I had suffered a very severe blow." Alon's automatic response and his default course of action was to berate himself. He judged and accused himself and his body which had betrayed him: "I nurtured my body and I worshipped it in endless hours at the gym, running on the beach, maintaining a healthy diet, meticulous hygiene, showing off my body to everyone but at the same times I defiled my body with drug addictions, endless screwing around and orgies -- and to cap it all, forgetting to put on a condom."

Nonetheless, in his very first phone conversation with the doctor who informed him of being a HIV positive carrier, Alon knew deep inside how he wished to handle his life as a carrier and in particular, how he did not want to conduct himself. He had seen carrier acquaintances shut themselves away, scared of going to the gay community clubs in order to avoid being talked about as carriers, scared of facing rejection (being told "no" on account of being carriers) and therefore living a solitary life of constant guilt. "I saw too many other carriers go back into the closet -- only this time it was the 'carrier closet' instead of the 'gay closet.' I had no intention of going back into any closet. My mission was not to blame anyone and especially not myself. My mission was to forgive myself."

1. **Identifying the "silver lining:"** (What are the benefits? What do we get? What do we learn?)

"An hourglass was placed in front of my eyes and forced them wide open." – I understood that life was short and that I needed and wanted to make it as fulfilling as possible as quickly as possible.

"There are worse things in life. I am not sick." – This is not cancer and this is not diabetes. This is merely being a carrier and there is an effective, well-known and organized preventive treatment.

"I no longer need to fear being infected." – The fear of being infected exists with all people and as far as I am concerned the worst has already happened. Ironically, this has opened up a lot of emotional space formally taken up by fear.

"Guilt does not get me anywhere." – From the very first moment I had this insight, an inner voice spoke very powerfully to me. That is why I never spent any time dealing with how I was infected or whether I was or was not aware when it happened.

"I was reinforced in the by the knowledge that I was a moral individual" – There was simply no way for me to conceal from my sexual partners that I am a carrier and even my body refused to deceive them by not cooperating with the act unless I came clean. I simply had no erection if I didn't.

2. **Identifying the "Why?"** (What are we missing? What is stuck / obstructed? What is not being implemented? What is striving to get out? What is being reflected upon us? Who is our mirror?)

Alon delved into the depths of his soul and came up with two significant insights: The first is related to love and the other is associated with rejection. "It turns out that I created this situation because I needed love. This body which I nurtured and supposedly loved, brought me men who loved my body much more than I loved it and it is only through them and through the way that they looked at me and desired me that I loved it and loved myself. However, this was not truly self-love. This was hollow and empty. The HIV, ironically, proved to be the key towards developing self-love."

One of the greatest difficulties associated with being a carrier is rejection, the fear of being rejected for being an HIV carrier. For Alon, the roots of rejection and absence of self-love were deeply rooted all throughout his childhood since he grew up with a harsh and critical father, a man who was verbally violent towards all of the family members, who lived under a regime of emotional terror. "My father constantly rejected me, never accepted me, criticized me and constantly cursed me. I never felt any love from him or felt wanted in any way." Understanding the sources of the constant rejection, understanding how a child growing up in the absence of love grows up to be a man who does not love himself and the understanding of how a child who is constantly criticized and berated eventually engages in constant self-criticism eventually helped Alon vent out the enormous pain of rejection and the anger trapped within him, opening the way to self-forgiveness and eventually forgiveness for his father as well. "I had no choice but to find myself anew within myself. I learned and understood in the tunnels of my soul that the way for self-acceptance is primarily through self-forgiveness. There is no more room for berating myself and so, in spite of all of the difficulties in being a carrier = rejection, once I forgave myself I learned to accept and love myself not in spite of my 'flaw' but thanks to this "flaw.""

3. **What to change?**

**Changing how we think:** (new perspectives on the situation)

"I am valuable, worthy and loved in spite of being an HIV carrier."

"The universe made me a carrier for my own supreme good." – It is only thanks to being infected that I learned to accept myself.

"There is no longer any room for the default choice of berating oneself. – I exorcise it and do not give it any place in my life. Today, there is plenty of space for a good hug and forgiveness.

"I want to live life more powerfully."

"I need to change my debauched lifestyle."

**Changing how we feel:** (What is the new emotion towards the situation? Does it include appreciation and thankfulness?)

"I love being made a carrier and the opportunity it brought to me and I am grateful towards it. I feel like I received a gift."

"I have no more fear of 'no.' I have no more fear of rejection." – The moment I feel valuable on the inside, there is no more room for fear. What others think of me is irrelevant because I feel complete.

**Changing what we do:** (How can we act differently? Behave differently? Respond differently? Speak differently?)

"I am a calmer man than I once was." – Being infected brought more serenity into my life.

"I learned not to judge myself or my environment." – Being a carrier opened my mind to the possibility of greater compassion and less judgments towards others.

"I embrace my past and future errors." – Without berating myself but with a good hug and wholehearted understanding that mistakes happen and that is how we learn."

"I stopped with the no holds barred debauchery." – I really geared down and look after myself and others more. I always wear a condom and no longer share my exploits in bed with the entire world. I placed limits on myself.

"I no longer get upset with little things that would have irritated me in the past." – I decided to have fun without all of the unnecessary stress. I take stuff to heart less and don't get offended as much

## *Time to get to work -- being our own psychologists...*

So after we read, learned, understood and saw illustrations of how this system was implemented and assisted others in various situations, obstructions and challenges, it is time to help ourselves, pull up our sleeves and delve deeper into our internal world. It is, in short, time to ask questions. It is time to reconnect with the spiritual perspective within us and to shine a light on the dark and painful places that are clamoring for attention and healing in the shape of the challenges that we face. It is time to grow into the next level of existence.

For your convenience the following pages condense and summarize the three parts that make up the trilogy method:

The first and second part – These are the early preliminary and theoretical parts.

The third part -- This is the practical part which asks the questions we must answer if we wish to help ourselves.

Find a quiet corner or some quiet time, put your cell phones on silent, take a few deep breaths in order to relax and calm down your system, go over the information condensed here, let it percolate and prepare the territory (on the mental and emotional level) and then ask yourselves these three questions.

Do not be disappointed if you do not receive immediate answers. Most of you will not get immediate answers. Do not be angry with yourselves if you cannot understand the full picture. Most of you will only figure out a small piece of the puzzle at a time. Do not be disappointed with yourselves if resistance results. Most of you will initiate a defense mechanism that will deny access to the heavily defended and fortified regions of your soul. Remember that therapy at a psychologist does not provide you with all the answers at a single meeting either. The most important thing is simply to begin asking these important questions. Repeatedly. Dare to reconnect to yourself and to all of the parts of which you, like everyone, is composed and most importantly persist at it!

**Set down in your diary a permanent weekly appointment, just as in a "real" therapy.**

**Treat this time as sacred, just as in a "real" therapy.**

**Listen to what arises from within, just like in a "real" therapy.**

If you are already going to some kind of therapeutic framework, bring the information that emerges with you and share it with your therapist – it will sharpen, focus and empower you and improve the effectiveness of the treatment itself.

Summary of the primary
# principles of the trilogy


**PART 1** The three parts of man


- Man is made up of three parts: The temporal body, the soul and the eternal spirit.

- The visual angle of the spirit: Eternal and immortal, a high vantage point that looks upon life from a bird's-eye view. It is concerned with the lessons our life is supposed to teach us. It acts from an existence of cosmic, non-linear, interdependent time where everything occurs simultaneously and no space-time limitations exist.

- The spirit is essentially a mixture of supreme grace, of universal harmony, of compassion, of love, of calm, of serenity, of acceptance and of a superior intellect that enables near automatic understanding of "Why things are as they are."

- If we compare the spirit to the Waze navigation application: It has all of the data regarding all of the possible routes we might take and it knows the destination for each of them. It does not interfere with our choices and merely offers us the optimal alternative given its analysis of all of the data.

- The spirit speaks in a small still voice and it is difficult for us to hear it in this noisy and chaotic world, particularly given our thick emotional defenses.

- The spirit is creative and varied in its approaches -- it has an infinite number of paths in which it can reach us and mark the way leading to our supreme good: It speaks to us through our feelings and sensations (shining a light on the inner dark), through manipulating situations in our external reality (opportunities for change and development), through dreams (guidance and messages that are transmitted through individualized symbolism), through pains and diseases (opportunities to discard which do not support the body and the soul), through hunches and intuitions (which motivate us to action even in the absence of a sufficient logical explanation), through inspiring ideas which "suddenly" appear in our head (in moments of "temporary shutdown" such as light rest, staring at the air, reflection, serenity or relaxation) and through powerful epiphanies of the heart (which bypass all sense and logic).

- Awareness of the sophisticated style of "speech" leads to recognition of our growth-delaying and growth-promoting mechanisms and to acceptance of the circumstances of life from understanding that they are imbued with a lesson which is meant to take us to the next step of our development.

- A spiritual man manages an ongoing and tri-directional communication between body, soul and spirit out of a desire to receive guidance, find the signs of this guidance, be exposed to the superior intellect of the spirit and to identify supportive probabilities and opportunities as they arise in his life.

- A man who develops spiritually develops both emotionally and in his consciousness while implementing the spiritual knowledge in the reality of his life and getting to know himself in all of the various layers of his soul.

## PART 2 The three premises

### The First Premise
*Opportunities arrive in disguise*

- We are not always aware of what we truly desire of ourselves, of others or of life itself.

- Our true desire is hidden beneath opportunities that arrive at our door. If we learn how to identify this desire, we will learn how to exploit these opportunities to the fullest.

- The reasons for preferring the known difficulties over an unfamiliar opportunity include: Negative emotions overwhelm reason and logic, we prefer to stick to the familiar, we are afraid of the unknown, our habits usually gain the upper hand and, critically, we fail to recognize the opportunities that arrive disguised in various costumes.

- The masks donned by the opportunities are cunning and can create considerable confusion since the opposite of what we seemingly want arrives. For example: We want to nurture and develop our courage and a terrifying lion arrives so that we will have the chance to overcome our fear and be brave.

- There is an "altitude gap" between the desires of the eternal spirit (which are independent of passions, urges and ego, are supreme and deal with the big picture and the master plan), to the desires of the temporal soul (grounded and dealing with the micro and everyday life). This gap in altitude can cause considerable frustration.

- The mechanism of disguise is the overlapping point of similarity between the seemingly opposed desires of the temporal soul and the eternal spirit and both make use of it.

- There is a meticulous planning and a sublime integration of both earthly and supreme reasons (a higher consciousness which understands "Why things are as they are") and which gives us the opportunity to choose differently, to change and be changed.

- Awareness of the sophisticated disguise mechanism of opportunities will help us accept the circumstances of our life as a journey of self-development that will bring us to a better place -- even if it looks and feels exactly the opposite.

## The Second Premise
*self-compassion instead of berating oneself*

- This premise is a chance to move on to examine the circumstances of our life and the places where we are stuck from a position of self-compassion rather than one of berating oneself.

- At some point in our lives, we have become the harshest judge of ourselves and we are berating, criticizing, belittling and not supporting ourselves.

- Throughout our lives, we have been criticized, we have been humiliated, we have been shamed and accused and at some point we have simply begun to believe all of these terrible things about ourselves. We believe that we deserve all the evil / difficulties / punishment / suffering we encounter.

- Until recent times, no awareness existed regarding the destructive consequences of words on emotions, behavior and the character of an individual.

- Conclusions, beliefs and perceptions through the neural pathways in our brain where they are repeatedly applied, become our "absolute truth" which operates us and becomes the lens through which we perceive and comprehend reality. We believe it.

- Self-compassion – It means that when we suffer, fail or feel unworthy, we treat ourselves with understanding and kindness rather than berating ourselves with self-criticism (or else suppressing, ignoring or fleeing the pain and the unpleasant feeling).

- Compassion is the way to answer the eternal question "Why are things the way they are?" and it is like the torch shining a light into a dark room and showing us the true shape of things.

- Examining challenging situations in our lives from a place of self-compassion also enables greater honesty and openness (which grants us the courage to dive into deeper layers) as well as the development of a spiritual perspective.

- Self-compassion gives birth to insights, which lead to acceptance of the situation. This enables us to undertake the change and progress beyond the obstruction or challenging situation.

## The Third Premise
*Every setback is an opportunity for growth*

- All things in the universe, large and small, grow and evolve, whether they are plants, animals, humans or the universe itself.

- In human beings, growth occurs in four parallel layers: *Physical growth* (growth-growing old-dying), *psychological growth* which is composed from two channels: *Mental growth* (learning to accumulate knowledge from the circumstances, experiences and events of our life) and *emotional growth* (learning how to relax, forgive and primarily open up our hearts to ourselves and the environment), *energetic growth* (learning how to raise and stabilize our frequency as much as possible since such a high frequency is accompanied by a positive feeling) and *spiritual growth* (combing the three other types of growth with the connection to the spirit -- our eternal and hidden part).

- *When we are* stuck, stand in place and do not develop, we get a little push from reality. Life will try to get us out of our comfort zone and will create for us situations, events and conditions that will force us to stop, reflect and change. We will be forced to grow.

- It is recommended you recite two supporting axioms daily: "*Whatever comes my way, comes to develop me.*" (Refers to situations reality throws at us) and "Whatever rises to the surface, rises on its way out." (Refers to negative emotions,) Together, they provide us with a cerebral and emotional understanding of what is happening to us and they help us reduce the emotional pain we feel.

- If we can take to heart the axiom that everything that happens to us is designed to help us evolve, we can transform the equation "failure = shame = pain" to the equation "failure = learning = growth" and thereby reduce our pain and expand our spiritual perspective.

- *Negative emotions and pain are like giant torches aimed inwards* inviting us to discover the painful story behind them. *In the first stage,* it will be easier for us to accept ourselves in this situation. *In the second stage,* we will ask questions so as to get direction to the place within us that is in pain and seeking a response. *In the third stage*, in order to release and purge that pain, we will feel it repeatedly and pass through it until it fades. This is a pain with a defined purpose and goal, a pain of stemming from release and a healing process.

- Cleaning up the particles of emotional waste within us, one particle at a time, transforms our worldview into a more positive one, as if we removed negative lenses from our eyes.

## PART 3 The three trilogy questions:

### The First Question
*Where is the silver lining in the cloud?*

- When we arc in pain, angry or suffering, we are on "the dark side of the moon" and we do not feel like leaving it or trying harder in order to see the "light" on the other side.

- The positive and joyful question "Where is the silver lining in the cloud?" is based on the assumption that every situation or event contains something good. This question forces us to be positive and to leave the negativity to which we are accustomed, forcing us to find our growth potential.

- Our supreme good is our "big picture" good that deals with the long-range and not the short, that deals with our growth and our development and that leaves the boundaries of the "me" entering into the territory of the "we."

- Our supreme good is quite often the exact opposite of our immediate good and this is frustrating and annoying, particularly when it is painful or when it is hard and we want it to just end and end now.

- The reality that we experience and perceive is not an objective reality but our personal-emotional interpretation that is based on our experience and character and it can blur reality or blind our eyes.

- The "oversensitivity – biased interpretation – bent reality" mechanism exists in most human beings in various intensities and shapes. It is not that we are the only ones who are screwed up; it is simply part of the human condition.

- The silver lining which we seek in the most difficult situations embodies our supreme good, objectivity and the two types of benefits that hard situations provide us with -- things we receive (a response to hidden or apparent needs, the development of desired or neglected character traits) and what we learn (important lessons, knowledge and experience or new capabilities).

## The Second Question
*why did we create the situation?*

- We are required to assume responsibility for the situation but we are not guilty or seeking to assign guilt. Rather, we are seeking the lower and supreme reasons leading to the desired change.

- On the one hand, we create our reality in three layers: The *physical level* (our consciousness impacts particles of matter and changes it), on the *physiological level* (the body responds biologically -- according to what an individual believes) and on the *psychological level* (the soul creates a reality that matches our thoughts and emotions).

- On the other hand, we cannot truly create everything we might desire due to lack of faith (we are essentially negative, living in the past and dominated by defense mechanisms), ruled by our subconscious (it is the part of our mind really running our lives) and the existence of supreme reasons (whatever is not part of our life script and which is not part of our destiny will not come to pass).

- In order to discover the subconscious, supreme and lower reasons for the situation we are in, it is recom- mended that:

1. We *calm down* the system.
2. We extend our antennas and seek out signs.
3. We identify and acknowledge *supportive probabilities and coincidences.*

- "The external world is a reflection of the inner world." – The outer reality of our lives is a reflection of the inner reality within us (internal aspects in our lives that are seeking a response).

- *Guiding questions* which might help us discover the "Why?"

  - *What are we missing*? Personal qualities, communication skills, a certain value.

  - *What is stuck*? What is not flowing? What is not progressing sufficiently or at all? Are we being stalled or are we stalling?

  - *What are we not fulfilling*? A childhood dream, an unrealized dream, a personal or social role to be fulfilled.

  - *What is seeking release*? What aspects of our soul are seeking attention, relief and healing? The obstructions as traffic signs that are pointing us at painful places that are ripe to release the pain.

  - *What does the situation reflect for us?* The thing within us that is crying out for help, attention and recognition or healing is reflected to us through various situations and people in our reality. The key for identification – whatever you see in the outer world, exists in the inner world as well.

  - *Our mirrors* – The people in our lives teach us about ourselves by reflecting to us something that is within us. The rule of the thumb is – *whoever is irritating and angering us is reflecting for us.*

- Understanding the "why?" (The lower reasons, conscious

and subconscious and the supreme reasons) *eases the introduction of the desired changes* in our lives from a place of acceptance, compassion and a deep desire for growth rather than from a place of conflict or self-hate.

## The Third Question
### *What can we change?*

- This practical question takes the theoretical insights of the first two questions and uses the details inside *the reality of our material life*, into our everyday lives that includes our thoughts, our emotions and our actions.

- *The key word is will* – We must want to change and be changed.

- If we want to change our situation, we must *assume responsibility* for it -- or its creation (and the understanding that we create the reality of our life for the most part without being aware of it), and for leaving it (and the specific actions leading us there).

- **Changing how we think**

- Changing how we perceive our situation is made possible through 1. Acting out of *self-awareness and separation* from the specific situation. 2. *Concentrating on the data*: A list of benefits, a list of supreme and lower, subconscious reasons that led to the formation of this situation and a list of reflections. The answers to these questions are in and of themselves the solutions. 3. *Listing new perceptions* (a combination of spiritual perceptions and our supernal good).

- **Changing how we feel**

- Our thoughts and emotions are interwoven, affect each other and are affected by each other. That is why we must change how we feel towards the situation by: 1. *Identifying and confessing the emotion.* 2. *A conscious wish* to change that emotion. 3. *Cleaning and draining the negative emotions* out of us. 4. *A true appreciation* of the opportunity presented to us by the situation in the form of thankfulness.

- *The way to make changes is from the inside outwards. That is the proper order of things.* The inner change we performed in our thoughts and our emotions is what enables an outer change in behavior.

- **Changing our actions**

- The stage where we move from words to actions, from inner changes to outer changes, with the *list of new actions.* What can we do differently? How can we behave differently? How can we react differently? How can we speak differently?

- Seeing the bigger picture from above, looking at the long-term, leaving the boundaries of "me," referring to our supreme good, our growth and the establishment of a mutually beneficial relationship with the part within us that knows what we are here to accomplish, will lead to a change in the reality of our lives, a better feelings, a sense of satisfaction and existential security and a rise in the frequency of the moments of happiness and joy in our lives.

*And now, time to ask the three questions:*


1.  **"WHERE IS THE SILVER LINING IN THE CLOUD?"**


What do we *benefit* from the situation?

______________________________________

______________________________________

______________________________________


What do we *receive* (attention to visible or hidden needs or the development of desired or neglected characteristics)?

______________________________________

______________________________________

______________________________________


What do we *learn* (important lessons, knowledge and experience or new capabilities)?

______________________________________

______________________________________

______________________________________

## 2. "Why did we create the situation?"

What are we missing? A personal quality, communication, a certain value.

___________________________________________

___________________________________________

___________________________________________

What is stuck / obstructed? What isn't flowing? What is not progressing at all or not enough? Are we stalling or being stalled?

___________________________________________

___________________________________________

___________________________________________

What are we *not fulfilling*? A childhood dream, an unfulfilled dream, a personal or social purpose.

___________________________________________

___________________________________________

___________________________________________

What is striving to be released? What hidden aspects of our soul are seeking attention, relief and healing? The obstructions are traffic signs aiming at the dark, painful areas in our soul prepared to release their pain.

_______________________________________________

_______________________________________________

_______________________________________________

*What does the situation reflect for us?* The thing inside us seeking help, attention, recognition or healing is reflected to us through people and situations in our reality. The key for identification – what you see outside also exists inside.

_______________________________________________

_______________________________________________

_______________________________________________

*Who are our mirrors?* The people in our life teach us about ourselves by reflecting for us something that is within us. The rule is – whoever *irritates and angers us reflects upon us.*

_______________________________________________

_______________________________________________

_______________________________________________

3. **"W**HAT CAN WE CHANGE?**"**

**Changing how we think**

Concentrating the data: Listing the benefits (what we receive and learn), a list of subconscious supreme and lower reasons and a list of reflections.

_______________________________________________

_______________________________________________

_______________________________________________

A list of new perceptions (combining spiritual perspectives and our supreme good).

_______________________________________________

_______________________________________________

_______________________________________________

**Changing how we feel**

1.  Identifying and confessing our emotions. What do we really feel?

_______________________________________________

_______________________________________________

_______________________________________________

2. A conscious wish to change this emotion. Are we really
   ready / mature / ready for a change?

_______________________________________________

_______________________________________________

_______________________________________________

3. Cleaning and draining the negative emotions out of
   us (through writing, guided imagination, conversations…).

_______________________________________________

_______________________________________________

_______________________________________________

4. A genuine appreciation of the opportunity in the form
   of thankfulness (can come at a later stage. It is a process).

_______________________________________________

_______________________________________________

_______________________________________________

**Changing our actions**

*Listing new actions:*

What can we do differently?

____________________________

____________________________

____________________________

How can we behave differently?

____________________________

____________________________

____________________________

How can we respond differently?

____________________________

____________________________

____________________________

How can we speak differently?

____________________________

____________________________

____________________________